I0440259

Seizure Free Addressing the Causes of Seizures Naturally

MELINDA CURLE

Copyright © 2013 Melinda Curle

All rights reserved.

DEDICATION

This book is dedicated to my parents who stood by me through thick and thin. They were very supportive when I was on medication, but also supported my journey to obtain optimal health and come off of it.

CONTENTS

ACKNOWLEDGMENTS

This book would not have been possible without the coaching from Alicia Dunams' <u>Bestseller in a Weekend course</u>. It gave me the motivation to put my story into words and share it with other people. It isn't perfect, but Alicia taught me the importance to setting goals and following through when you write a book.

I am very grateful for my family, who lived through the intricacies of my seizures and still supported me.

1 INTRODUCTION

Seizures are complex problems that affect two percent of the population. It is unfortunate for those who suffer from seizures that doctors schedule visits for only about fifteen minutes in length. That is only enough time to do a neurological examination, ask how the patient is doing and write a prescription for medication. There is rarely any time for discussion to take place regarding the cause. In my experience, any discussion of the cause of my seizures was brushed off and I was given the answer of, "We don't know." That is convenient for the doctor and scary for the patient. What is currently happening is that since the doctors don't really know, they are prescribing medication to suppress the symptoms. They briefly mention that the drugs can damage your liver and that you probably shouldn't get pregnant while taking some of them... I couldn't help but think, "Don't I need my liver? What is going to happen when my liver is damaged? What then?" My concerns about the cause were never really

1

addressed by doctors because the importance of keeping me seizure free was the top priority during the fifteen minute doctor's visits.

This book was written to help people diagnosed with epilepsy naturally improve their seizure control; whether their goal is to complement their medication or replace their medication. There are some things which will enhance seizure control naturally that you can do every day. It took me years to sort through some of the things that would calm down the nervous system; the things that reportedly worked – but no one understood why – and I discovered the seizure-free program that is working for me now.

Seizures instill fear in you. One thing that I learned from becoming an entrepreneur is that action replaces fear. Many people with seizures are living in fear of having another seizure. My seizures were mostly controlled with medication and I only experienced a few random seizures whenever I forgot to take a dose. What I did have fears about were; losing my driver's license, someone else calling an ambulance and me not having the health insurance to pay for my medications. I was always afraid that I would go into debt because of the cost of my disease. I realized after two decades of living with epilepsy that you could do things to minimize your chances of having a seizure. When you take actions everyday that are known to help prevent seizures, your mind can be at peace, knowing that you are doing everything that you can to optimize your health. Your body has an amazing ability to heal itself. Optimizing your health will enhance not only your overall health, but your seizure control as well. The fear that you were feeling because of seizures will diminish over time.

Your neurologist may already tell you to exercise; eat a healthy diet and reduce stress; there are many ways to accomplish those three things, but not all of them will help prevent seizures. When you understand how these things impact your seizure control and the correct way to implement them, you will start to notice an overall change in your health and a lessening of your number of seizures. It is unfortunate that over the years the definition of a healthy diet has changed back and forth so many times. Just during my lifetime, I've seen eggs go from 'good for you' to' bad for you' and back again a number of times. Reducing stress is not as simple as it sounds and there are multiple forms of exercises to choose from. Which one is going to have the biggest impact on your seizure control?

This book explains the current trends in seizure treatment, so you can understand what a neurologist will do when you go to his office. It then delves into the main causes of seizures, so you will have an idea of the conditions that are required before a seizure can occur inside your brain. I review the benefits that come from naturally addressing the main causes of seizures; even if you have some seizures that are triggered by other causes. I also explain in this book the prevention strategies that I have integrated into my daily life to address the causes of seizures naturally, and finally I talk about some of the major challenges that are faced by

3

people with seizures and a few ways to conquer them.

This book also was written to share my experiences and my journey with epilepsy. I have already received criticism from people who embrace the Western medical approach to their seizures. A decade ago, I would have criticized someone who shunned the medical drugs that I was taking, because I felt that they worked and I didn't have any idea of what else to do. In fact, I was pretty convinced that my medication was the best and was shocked to hear from a classmate of mine who was suffering from seizures that the medication didn't work for her.

This book was also written to help other people understand the challenges that go along with epilepsy. I wrote this book to bring awareness about epilepsy and help empower people who are suffering. It is nice to get to know other people who have the condition and give them support, but for the most part, our condition is hidden. The drug companies don't really address epilepsy that well because the brain isn't as understood as other organs in the body.

2 TRENDS IN SEIZURE TREATMENT

Currently, when you go to the doctor after you've had a seizure, the doctor will conduct a neurological examination. This usually includes touching your finger to your nose and then back and forth to the doctor's finger. I've done it dozens of times and now it is starting to annoy me. The doctor will also schedule you for an electroencephalogram EEG and an MRI (magnetic resonance image) if it is your first seizure. The EEG is looking to see how much electrical activity is in your brain at the time. This gives the doctor a snapshot of what is going on during normal activity. The doctor may decide to prescribe anticonvulsants for you right away, or wait until you have had a second seizure before putting you on them. The MRI is to check out the structure of your brain and determine if there is a brain tumor that is causing the seizures. If there isn't, you probably won't have very many more MRI's done. This is the most common approach, especially for juvenile myoclonic epilepsy or any type of epilepsy that doesn't have comorbidity, or any type of seizure that has occurred that doesn't have some direct sort of cause such as a blow to the head, a virus or any other pre-existing disease. For example, my sister is a diabetic who had a seizure; but no tests were done because they attributed it to low blood sugar.

The doctor will likely prescribe a medication after a second unprovoked seizure. There are plenty of anticonvulsants available for doctors to choose from today. Depakote, Tegretol, Lamictal, Zonegram, Keppra and Vilpat are commonly prescribed anticonvulsants. I'm sure that there are many more that the pharmaceutical companies are developing. The funding of research for epilepsy usually goes towards developing new medications. Doctors tend to trust medication because there is research behind the effectiveness of medication. Rarely will someone research a technique for treatment that doesn't make him or her money. Research itself is expensive.

If your treatment choice is to take prescription drugs, it is very important to understand what you are about to take. Dilantin is the oldest anticonvulsant that I know about. Thousands of people have taken it – and the side effects are well known. Some doctors prefer to prescribe newer drugs that have fewer reported side effects. This is actually misleading. I fell for it twice. I switched from two drugs to one, Lamictal, when I wanted to just be taking one drug because it didn't have as many side effects. The reason that it didn't have as many side effects is that it hadn't been out long enough for them to be reported. As time went on, a more serious side effect emerged. When you switch medications you are trading one side effect from another because instead of being constantly drowsy, I started having episodes of double vision and vertigo that would occur spontaneously. These were often worse than the seizures because I was conscious. Keep this in mind when opting for a newer drug. You are choosing something with unreported side effects. At the time, doctors told me the only side effect of Lamictal was a deadly rash and we would know immediately if the rash appeared and they could then take me off of the drug. Now, almost two decades later, Lamictal has a long list of side effects. It is unlikely that you will experience every single side effect, but it is important to understand the side effects. The double vision wasn't a listed side effect when I experienced it. I went to an optometrist to get my eyes checked out, not realizing that I was experiencing a side effect of my anticonvulsant. I thought I was going crazy when my eyes checked out fine.

The medications that I tried were Depakote and Tegretol, Lamictal and Keppra. While they do work for me, I decided that the control wasn't complete and I was still dealing with side effects from the medication. Sometimes I felt like the side effects were worse than the seizures. I wasn't having daily seizures, so I also kind of felt like it was wasteful to be taking medication every single day when my seizures weren't occurring every single day. What scared me, though, was missing a medication dose and having a seizure. My seizure control was dependent on that dose of medication. One time when I was on the mail-order pharmacy plan in college, my medication didn't come on time. I hoped that it would show up in my mailbox that day – but it didn't – and missing that one dose led to a seizure.

There are some things that you should be concerned about when taking anticonvulsants, or any medication for that matter. There is no shortage of lawsuits. What will happen when you become dependent on a drug and someone else sues the pharmaceutical company and they have to stop producing it? What happens when you start experiencing the devastating side effects? You need to ask yourself how long you can put up with the side effects and trade one symptom for another. This is a question that doctors don't address very well. Their answer usually is, "Can you live with it?" or, "We can try another medication." The reality is that all seizure medications have a side effect. They are all altering your chemistry in some way to reduce the electrical activity in your brain and prevent a seizure.

Surgery

Surgery is another trend in the treatment of seizures. When the doctors look at candidates for surgery, they are looking at people who have a focus for their seizures. They cut out a part of the brain that exhibits a lot of electrical activity and hope that will eliminate the cause of seizures. For many people, it works. My first college roommate had the epilepsy surgery and didn't have seizures after that. I was a little jealous because I had to remember to take my medication every day or I would end up having a seizure. Unfortunately, I haven't kept in touch with her over the years to find out if she is seizure free to this day. There are many downsides to this treatment. You do lose part of your brain. While your brain does learn to rewire itself in order to compensate for the missing portion, you may lose some function in your body. There is always going to be a risk; whatever treatment you chose. I have read some posts online about people who had the surgery, but years later their seizures returned. Removing a portion of the brain doesn't change the conditions that caused the seizure in the first place, but it does remove the area of the brain where the seizures start; and that will eliminate seizures for that person.

Surgery is extremely expensive. Many people raise money and ask loved ones to donate for the surgery. This also creates a burden on the health insurance companies. While you have paid into the system, everyone else who is paying into the health insurance system is likely to have his or her premiums incrementally raised if enough people take advantage of this type of seizure prevention strategy. Because it is so very cost-prohibitive, I highly recommend implementing the seizure prevention strategies that are natural to see how much improvement that you can have without having surgery.

Diets

Epilepsy has been treated with fasting since Hippocrates and Galen. Physicians at the beginning of the 20th century also tried treating epilepsy with fasting. Bernard Macfadden, Hugh Conklin, Dr. McMurray and others reported that many of their patients were never afflicted with seizures after completing a 21-day fast, particularly if followed by a low carbohydrate diet. The problem is that one can not fast forever and often the seizures returned when the patients ended the fast. In 1921 it was discovered that fasting changes body metabolism. The liver uses body fat to produce substances called ketone bodies which can cross the blood-brain barrier and provide the body with energy. The brain normally uses glucose as an energy source, but during fasting, glucose is not available. It was believed that the ketone bodies stopped the seizure. Therefore, the diet that produced ketones was created. It is known as the ketogenic diet.

The ketogenic diet is an option that is often offered to young children who don't respond to medication. It severely restricts carbohydrates and proteins and replaces them with fat. The classic ketogenic diet provides a four to one ratio of fat to the combined weight of carbohydrate and protein, which is called a ketogenic ration. Meals consist primarily of butter, eggs, heavy cream and very small amounts of non-starchy vegetables and fruit. Supplements must be taken because the diet does not provide all the nutrients that the body needs. The down side to the ketogenic diet is that it is very intensive. Food is measured and carbohydrates are restricted. There are plenty of ketogenic diet success stories. Most of them are young children. The Mayo Clinic reported that initial use of

the diet produced seizure control in 95% of patients,
with 60% becoming seizure free. (Campbell-McBride
80-81) When children are on a diet, they often feel
isolated and left out at birthday parties or during
lunchtime at school. My diabetic sister resented all the
alternative "treats" that were given to her instead of the
full fat and full sugar version. Getting all the right
nutrients can be tough on this limited calorie diet. When
I look through some of the food recommendations, I
cringe; because they don't seem that healthy to me.
However, it does help some people become seizure free.

There is another diet that is prescribed to treat
seizures; the Modified Atkins Diet for Seizures. This
diet is a bit easier to follow and I have tried it. The
ketogenic ratio in the Modified Atkins Diet is much
simpler because it just restricts the number of
carbohydrates that you eat in a day. It places no limits
on protein and calories and can be done without
dieticians or hospital stays. However, you are on a
severely restricted amount of carbohydrates. For me, it
was 30 carbohydrates per day. These diets focus on
putting the body into ketosis, which tricks the body into
thinking that it is starving and that it doesn't have
enough energy for seizures – the glucose that is required
for seizures just isn't available. For some people it
works well. I did try out the Modified Atkins Diet for
Seizures, but despite staying strictly on 30 carbohydrates
per day and depriving myself of fruit, I ended up having
a couple of seizures. I decided to keep searching for
answers as I wasn't convinced at all that my seizures

11

were caused by food. In fact, I highly doubted that they were related to the foods that I ate because prior to diagnosis, I was a pretty liberal eater. I had tried out a bunch of different diets and still had seizures on them. I'm not claiming that diets won't help, because for some people simply changing their diet eliminates the seizures. However, for me, it wasn't the answer. Eating healthier is always recommended.

Dr. Natasha Campbell-McBride, who is a neurologist and the author of *Gut and Psychology Syndrome*, also known as the GAPS diet, created a diet to address the nutritional deficiencies, which can be found in people with epilepsy, as well as limiting the number of seizures by limiting the carbohydrates in the body. I recommend her book because I found it fascinating and tried the GAPS diet for eight months. While it didn't eliminate my seizures, I felt that my body benefited from eating healthier and I learned the ways that an abnormal gut flora can impact your overall health. Her treatment of seizures focuses on reducing the level of toxicity in the body and addressing nutritional deficiencies.

As you can see, there are lots of ways to become seizure free if one of them doesn't work for you. For some people, surgery is an option and they are comfortable with the risks. Other people wouldn't dream of changing their lifestyle and eating habits and prefer to live with the side effects. My goal shifted from being seizure free on medication to having optimal health. It really doesn't matter if you are seizure free if your health is so bad in other areas. I was getting autoimmune diseases, seeing double and having vertigo. I had to get optimal health to start enjoying life again.

The reality is that your body changes from moment to moment. You are more at risk of seizures during certain time periods; after over-eating and if you have poor sleep patterns. Sometimes the seizure medication builds up in your system and your body starts to need more of it in order to produce the same effect. Unfortunately, it also increases the side effects that you have to deal with. You must determine if living with those side effects and that cycle is something that you want to continue throughout your life. For some people it will be acceptable to live with the side effects from the medication. Other people will determine that the seizures aren't bad enough to warrant taking medication that produces side effects. I experienced some horrific side effects and determined that they were worse than the seizures.

3 CAUSES OF SEIZURES

I remember being a scared thirteen year old who had experienced a few tonic clonic seizures. Sitting in Dr. Potolicchio's office, I asked him, "What is the cause of my seizures?" He was kind and answered in a funny way, but one that I still remember to this day. Dr. Potolicchio said, "It is idiopathic. That means, we're idiots and don't know the cause." That really broke the ice for me and helped me feel comfortable with him. I trusted his frankness and humor. Through my teenage years as I saw him scratch his head and just incrementally raise my dose and add another medication, I thought that being a neurologist was probably the easiest thing in the world – you are just guessing and checking which medication works. However, today I strongly feel that Dr. Potolicchio's statement regarding the cause of seizures is inaccurate.

What I found upsetting was the thought that if
something is idiopathic and you have no idea what
causes it, what are you doing prescribing a medication
for it? The medication is going to do something to the
person's body. Shouldn't there be some need to address
a cause? Doctors are creating a dependence on
medication to suppress the symptom of seizures instead
of addressing the cause of the seizures. They actually do
know that they are only suppressing the symptoms, but it
is the only solution that they have. They are trained in
medicine and they read the medical studies from the
pharmaceutical companies.

Main Cause of Seizures

There are thousands of individual triggers; and that
is one of the problems with seizure treatment. When
you identify sixty different things that will cause
seizures in different people, it is easier to find a powerful
chemical that will simply suppress the symptoms rather
than have someone try to avoid or eliminate all the
different foods, toxins and activities from their lives.
However, there is one thing that will reliably trigger the
brain's seizure activity in people who are prone to
seizures, those with epilepsy and even a person who has
never had a seizure in their life. That would be
hyperventilation. This is not really even discussed
during the visits with the neurologist. They don't teach
you how to address chronic hyperventilation. They may
not even realize that it impacts your overall health.

Doctors are aware of two main underlying causes that will induce epileptic seizure activity in the brain. What? Your doctor didn't tell you this? No, mine didn't either. It was briefly mentioned, but not really discussed. The EEG test gives you some insight into what doctors know will trigger seizure activity. The EEG begins with a period of hyperventilation and flickering lights. Doctors know that these two things reliably trigger electrical activity in most people, even people without seizures. Hyperventilation will trigger seizure activity in the brain. That is what they are looking for during an EEG. That is the reason that they have you hyperventilate. Some people who have seizures can actually hyperventilate and cause a seizure. The photic stimulation is the blinking lights. This is very irritating, and if the seizures are starting in that part of the brain, it will show an increase of electrical activity.

Under normal conditions all electrical signals that are traveling along the nerve cells are related to important and objective processes, for example – doing the work of the senses, memory, analysis, logic, decision-making, and the involuntary and voluntary muscle movements. An electrical signal travels from one nerve cell to the next when the voltage or strength of the signal is high enough. It should be no less than a certain threshold value. This threshold directly relates to the seizure threshold. The normal value for the threshold of excitability is roughly fifty microvolts in humans, although individual thresholds vary.

When the seizure threshold is high, the electrical signals are transmitted normally. With normally transmitted electrical signals, adaptation and self-improvement are the normal outcomes in these people. For the normal outcome to happen, it is crucial that when the neuronal signals are transmitted that the signals are transmitted and facilitated through the network of nerve cells, and irrelevant signals become hampered and do not interfere with the normal work of the senses: memory, solution-making, decision-making and feedback. For people with epilepsy, memory, solution-making, feedback and decision-making can be impaired when they aren't having seizures because of this lowered seizure threshold. When the seizure threshold becomes too low, the irrelevant signals can be amplified and disruption of the entire system may occur. This happens when abnormal changes occur during breathing. The balance of oxygen and carbon dioxide becomes low in the brain. The most common abnormality with abnormal breathing is arterial hypocapnia, or low carbon dioxide, and cell hypoxia, low oxygen in the brain. Chronic hyperventilation is the key cause for both of these conditions. (http://www.normalbreathing.com/d-seizure-threshold.php)

While you may not think that you are hyperventilating, your breathing rate is probably faster than it needs to be for optimal health. In fact, according to Artour Rakhimov, founder of the Normalbreathing.com website, most modern individuals are breathing at a rate that is twice as much as an optimal level. This will impact your health in many different ways. If a certain organ isn't getting enough oxygen, it may start to shut down or produce less. In the brain, it creates an environment where the brain isn't functioning optimally and there is a greater chance of having a seizure.

How does this affect seizures? The seizure threshold, or excitability of the nerve cells, is very sensitive to oxygen and carbon dioxide. A low level of carbon dioxide will cause abnormal excitability of nerve cells. Studies have proven that hyperventilation "leads to spontaneous and asynchronous firing of neurons." Therefore, when we hyperventilate or breathe more than the norm, oxygen and carbon dioxide levels in the cells become abnormally low. This can cause irrelevant or weak electrical signals to be strengthened and relayed through the brain and interfere with the normal signals which are reducing the seizure threshold.

Chronic hyperventilation is an underlying cause of different types of seizures. Numerous medical studies prove that hyperventilation reliably increases the electrical activity in people with epilepsy and patients suffering from seizures. When I had my last EEG, the technician told me that even people who don't have seizures could have seizure activity in their brain during hyperventilation. Hyperventilation increases the electrical activity in your brain and when it gets to a certain point, you will have a seizure.

In my opinion, doctors aren't prescribing changing

the way that you breathe because they don't feel that you have control over it. It is under the control of your autonomic nervous system. While you don't have control over it during the nighttime, there are some things that you can do about it. In fact, during the day you can retrain your body to lower the rate at which you breathe. You can also retrain your body to breath with your diaphragm so that the lower chambers of your lungs receive oxygen.

Individuals report stress as another main cause of seizures. Stress varies so much between individuals that it is difficult to address. Additionally, it isn't psychological stress that causes the seizures; it is how the body is reacting to the stress. When we have stress, often we end up hyperventilating, or breathing shallowly and rapidly. Stress can cause disrupted sleep conditions and that can put the patient into a state of rapid breathing. Stress is more or less a common trigger. However, knowing that it is a common trigger helps us to address it naturally and prevent seizures.

There are many factors that can influence the seizure threshold in addition to hyperventilation. However, if you eliminate hyperventilation you will reduce the influence that those factors have on your body. Low blood glucose levels can trigger and prolong seizures. Chronic hyperventilation worsens general blood sugar control, increasing the symptoms of reactive hypoglycemia. Low blood carbon dioxide can induce vasoconstriction and cause a spasm of the carotid artery that can be an aggravating factor. (Fainting following hyperventilation is partially based on the same effect: breathing too shallowly and frequently will decrease the glucose availability for the brain.)

Reduced brain oxygenation due to chest breathing, suppressed Bohr Effect and vasoconstriction is an additional factor that will increase the acidity of brain cells. This can intensify abnormal electrical activity and lower the seizure threshold even more.

It is safe to say that the main cause of seizures is arterial hypocapnia, or a low carbon dioxide level in the arterial blood. The main effects of hypocapnia caused by hyperventilation are an increased excitability of nerve cells that lowers seizure threshold; causes a reduction in brain-oxygen level and increased cellular acidity; reduces the amount of glucose available for the brain and worsens blood-glucose control; increases muscular tension and worsens the ability to resist stress due to a weakened immune system.
(http://www.normalbreathing.com/d-seizures-cause.php)

If someone with epilepsy can normalize their arterial carbon dioxide level and eliminate the cause of seizures by learning how to breathe no more than the international norm for breathing, the symptoms of epilepsy should disappear. This is the main thing that has helped me control my seizures naturally. The other thing that you can proactively do to reduce your chances of seizures is to reduce common seizure triggers. A friend of mine discovered her triggers, avoids them like the plague and has been able to control her seizures without medication as well.

If you are interested in reading the studies that support the claims I am making, I have included some of the abstracts for you. This will give you an idea of what was occurring during the study, if the patients had a form of epilepsy similar to yours, and if you feel that it can benefit you.

"Studies designed to determine the effects produced by hyperventilation on nerve and muscle have been consistent in their finding on increased irritability" Brown EB, *Physiological effects of hyperventilation*, Physiological Reviews 1953 October, Vol. 33 No. 4; p. 445-471.

Fried R, Rubin SR, Carlton RM, and Fox MC,
Behavioral control of intractable idiopathic seizures: I. Self-regulation of end-tidal carbon dioxide,
Psychosom Med. 1984 Jul-Aug;46(4):315-31.

Eleven women and seven men with moderate to severe chronic hyperventilation and idiopathic seizures refractory to therapeutic serum levels of anticonvulsant medication were given diaphragmatic respiration training with percent end-tidal CO_2 biofeedback. The training had a rapid correcting effect on their respiration, making it comparable to that of 18 asymptomatic control subjects. Ten of the seizure-group subjects were in the study at least 7 months and following treatment, 8 showed EEG power spectrum "normalization", restoration of cardio-respiratory synchrony (RSA), and **their seizure frequency and severity were significantly reduced.**

Neurol Neurochir Pol. 1981 Sep-Dec; 15 (5-6):545-52. [Effect of physical exertion on seizure discharges in the EEG of epilepsy patients] [Article in Polish] Horyd W, Gryziak J, Niedzielska K, Zielinski JJ.

Abstract: The purpose of this study was to establish the effect of moderate exercise on EEG tracings in young epileptics. The model of graded exercise was a 15-minute workout on a cycle ergometer. The effect of the exercise on the pattern of a simultaneously recorded EEG was compared with the effect of 3-minute hyperventilation. After testing a control group of 20 young subjects without evidence of organic brain damage; or with this damage causing no epilepsy, another group of 43 epileptics was studied. In none of these patients the intensity of changes in EEG increased during the exercise, but evident EEG differences could be detected during different stages of the exercise in 28 patients with significant generalized discharges. It was found that during the exercise in nearly all patients the number of discharges decreased, while during hyperventilation it increased. In 10 patients in this group a repeated rise in the number of discharges was observed immediately after the exercise, which was connected usually with greater fatigue after the exercise. In the light of these results the authors concluded that **moderate exercise inhibits seizure activity in EEG, contrary to hyperventilation, which increases these changes**.

The following study relates to absence seizures. My seizures were grand mal seizures, but some people suffer from more mild seizures. The conclusion regarding hyperventilation is highlighted.

Paediatr Drugs. 2001;3(5):379-403. Treatment of typical absence seizures and related epileptic syndromes. Panayiotopoulos, CP. Department of Clinical Neurophysiology and Epilepsies, St Thomas' Hospital, London, England.
tom.panayiotopoulos@gstt.sthames.nhs.uk

Typical absences are brief (seconds) generalised seizures of sudden onset and termination. They have 2 essential components: clinically, the impairment of consciousness (absence) and, generalised 3 to 4Hz spike/polyspike and slow wave discharges on electroencephalogram (EEG). They differ fundamentally from other seizures and are pharmacologically unique. Their clinical and EEG manifestations are syndrome-related. Impairment of consciousness may be severe, moderate, mild or inconspicuous. This is often associated with motor manifestations, automatisms and autonomic disturbances. Clonic, tonic and atonic components alone or in combination are motor symptoms; myoclonia, mainly of facial muscles, is the most common. The ictal EEG discharge may be consistently brief (2 to 5 seconds) or long (15 to 30 seconds), continuous or fragmented, with single or multiple spikes associated with the slow wave. The intradischarge frequency may be constant or may vary (2.5 to 5Hz). **Typical absences are easily precipitated by hyperventilation in about 90% of untreated patients...**

More evidence to support the theory that hyperventilation is at the root cause of seizures continues:

J ECT. 2008 Sep;24(3):195-8. Moderate hyperventilation prolongs electroencephalogram seizure duration of the first electroconvulsive therapy. Sawayama E., Takahashi M., Inoue A., Nakajima K., Kano A., Sawayama T., Okutomi T., Miyaoka H. Department of Psychiatry, Kitasato University School of Medicine, Sagamihara, Japan. enami@kitasato-u.ac.jp

Abstract; Although it is controversial that seizure duration can influence the efficacy of electroconvulsive therapy (ECT), a missed or brief seizure is considered less effective ECT. Of the background in the practice of ECT, **hyperventilation may augment the seizure duration**. To elucidate these hypotheses, we performed double-blind randomized controlled trials for 19 patients. They were divided into 2 groups, according to the end-tidal pressure of carbon dioxide (ETCO2): The moderate hyperventilation group with ETCO2 of 30 mm Hg and the normal ventilation group with ETCO2 of 40 mm Hg. ECT was performed under general anesthesia with propofol and suxamethonium. During ECT electroencephalogram (EEG) and electromyogram were recorded. The Global Assessment of Functioning scores were also analyzed before and after 6 sequential ECT. **The moderate hyperventilation group showed a significant increase in EEG seizure duration in the first treatment compared with the normal ventilation group ($P < 0.05$)...**

Common seizure triggers

According to the epilepsy foundation, there is no identifiable cause of seizures. Head injuries or lack of oxygen during birth may damage the delicate electrical system in the brain. Other causes may include brain tumors, genetic conditions and lead poisoning. Some factors include ingesting substances, hormone fluctuations, stress, sleep patterns and photosensitivity.

According to a friend of mine, one of the main seizure triggers that she experienced was gluten. Her body would react to gluten. Her biggest challenge was being around people who consumed gluten. This actually makes sense. Gluten requires a lot out of your digestive system and will lower the oxygen levels for a time while you are digesting it. If you are chronically hyperventilating, your brain's seizure threshold is probably lower while eating this food; and eating it pushes the threshold even lower, triggering a seizure.

In an online poll from seizuretracker.com, the two most common seizure triggers are stress and irregular sleep. Stress can cause hyperventilation as a physiological response, so it makes sense that eliminating your chronic hyperventilation would get rid of stress seizures. Irregular sleep is a tricky trigger to address. However, if you are able to improve the quality of your sleep and ensure normal breathing during sleep, you should be able to reduce your seizures.

As quoted by Epilepsy.com, some seizure triggers include: a specific time of day, sleep deprivation, fevers or other illnesses, flashing bright lights, alcohol or drug use, stress, hormonal changes, not eating well, low blood-sugar levels, specific foods and the use of certain medications.
(http://epilepsy.com/epilepsy/seizure_triggers) Some of these will be easy for you to avoid during your lifetime. You can choose to avoid drugs and alcohol. You can choose healthy, unprocessed whole foods very easily. Some things aren't as easy to address; such as the hormone fluctuations or the time of day. In those instances, implementing my seizure prevention strategies may work well for you.

I created an informal Facebook survey to discover the seizure triggers that affect people, and posted it online. Here are the results of my informal online survey about seizure triggers.

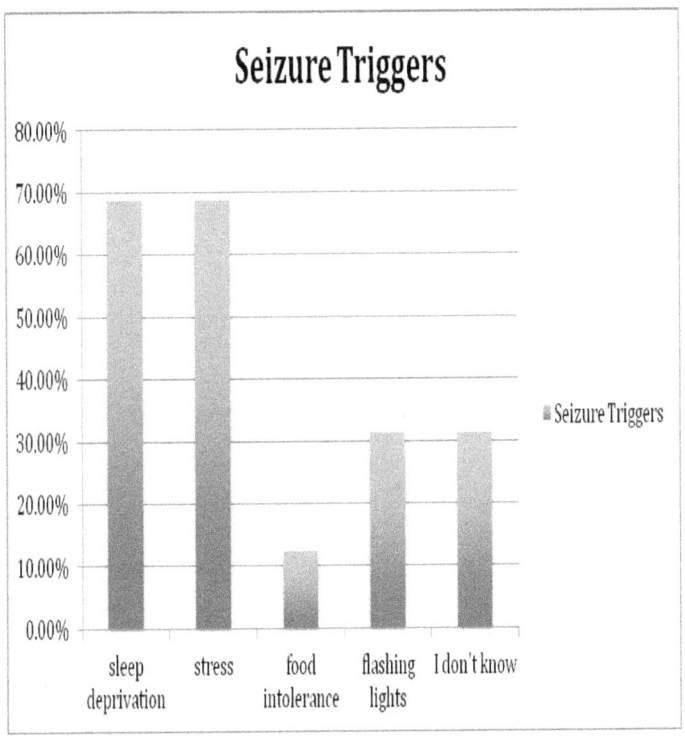

4 BENEFITS TO TREATING SEIZURES NATURALLY

Many doctors are very opposed to people with epilepsy eliminating their medication. There are also many individuals who are on medication who feel that really helps them and oppose even the idea of not taking seizure medication. The reason is that they simply don't understand seizures and what causes them. They place their trust in prescription medication which has a track record for reducing seizures. What people don't understand is that while the people with epilepsy may be seizure free, they are living with side effects and paying a huge price. Addressing seizures naturally has its benefits, but it does require effort. Keep these benefits in mind while you are implementing my exercise and breathing techniques into your own daily life. Knowing the benefits will help keep you focused on regularly putting into practice the prevention strategies.

First and foremost, you don't have to worry about whether or not you remembered to purchase your medication. You aren't concerned with whether you took it on time that morning or forgot. Often, I would find myself thinking about my morning routine and perhaps remembering the day before and assuming that I took my medication. I had a pillbox and when I examined the pillbox the next day, I would realize that I hadn't taken it. It was a common occurrence. I would always be wondering, "Did I take my medication?" There were a few times when I had to race back home from work to take the pill. When you learn to address seizures naturally, you can eliminate this worry from your life.

Financially, you won't be as burdened by epilepsy if you start to change your lifestyle to be less conducive to seizures. I remember coming out of college and living with my parents because I couldn't afford my disease. It was costing them about a thousand dollars a month. My parents paid for my medical expenses as a way to lower their tax bracket. While I'm grateful for that, I realize that not everyone has parents who can afford to do that. I couldn't afford my health insurance and the two medications that I was on. I really limited myself in the activities that I chose to do because they had to be safe and inexpensive. An ambulance ride ends up costing the person with seizures roughly $500; usually more because that is after the health insurance co-payment. I always worried that I would have an unexpected ambulance bill to pay; and occasionally I did. It just wasn't fair, because I would ask not to take the ride, but if they arrived before I'd regained consciousness, I would be taken to the emergency room to get checked out anyway. Financially, seizures were draining me. Staying medicated kept me classified as epileptic to health insurers.

Can your health afford to continue taking the seizure medication? When I used to figure out budgets and ways to afford medication, health insurance and unexpected emergency room visits, they were never accurate, and I usually ended up with other medical expenses and other medical problems. Anticonvulsants lowered the calcium uptake in my blood. I knew that was a side effect, but never imagined that I would end up with two root canals and two cracked teeth before the age of 30. The impact that poor eating habits, which my doctor never addressed, and prescription drugs had on my dental health was devastating. I'm not the only one who ended up with deteriorated dental health due to prescription medication. I spoke with a co-worker just the other day who had epilepsy and was happy with his seizure control, but he commented that he had cavities in every one of his teeth and his gums were receding and swollen because of the Dilantin. He commented that he would rather live with the side effects and was rather happy with the seizure control that the drug was giving him. I did notice that he spoke slower than the average person. He also repeatedly asked me questions that I had answered. Some people may attribute that to his age, but I knew that was probably similar to what my mother was talking about when she told me I was 'slower' when I was on medication. I started eating healthier and eliminated my medication and haven't had a cavity since.

Anticonvulsants cause other problems. My thyroid was always testing low when I was taking the anticonvulsants. I never had symptoms of hypothyroidism prior to taking anticonvulsants or after coming off anticonvulsants. I'm not sure if there was a correlation there or not, but I spent years visiting an endocrinologist and taking synthroid. That added an extra expense to my already low budget.

Eliminating medication from your life is very empowering. I chose to do it despite my doctor's warnings and the risk that I could have a seizure because I knew that I could no longer depend on the drugs. (Even when I took them daily, I would have an occasional seizure that would eliminate my driving privileges and make me feel horrible.) It is empowering because now I know that I am in control. I know that there is something that I can do when I start feeling an aura. Now I actually feel an aura instead of going straight into the seizure without feeling it because I'm was too medicated. I know I have to do certain activities every day for seizure prevention. My overall health is better and I feel like I can actually accomplish things now. I feel empowered!

Eliminating medication and treating seizures naturally requires that you obtain optimal health. Epilepsy is a disease that has been created in your body through unhealthy circumstances; just like heart disease, diabetes, eczema and asthma. Your body isn't functioning like it should and the best way to get it back to normal is going to be through the correct form exercise and eating healthy foods. Once you have reached an optimal level of health, the risk of seizures decreases greatly. You also enjoy the benefits of more restful sleep and more energy. I've noticed that I have clearer thinking and better skin. I'm starting to do more things and be more productive. Becoming free from the grasp of medication enables you to live a healthier life. You will have the mental abilities to focus better. You lower your chances of depression, which often occurs due to having seizures. It enables you to experience more joy. Seizure medications are often used to treat depression. They stabilize your moods in such a way that you don't experience highs and lows. I often felt numb to emotions when I was on two anticonvulsants. While I didn't really experience depression, I also didn't feel much elation and joy. Coming off medication, I feel like I have much more control over my emotions and experience a lot more joy.

When you eliminate medication from your life, you are no longer swapping one symptom for another that is easier to live with. Due to the fact that there are chemicals in the medication and you take it internally, you are impacting your whole body. You are not just suppressing the brain. There are side effects because you cannot get the chemicals to the one part of the brain without them going through your entire blood stream. There will be trade offs in your health when you choose to take medication to treat your seizures. These can come in the form of dizziness, double vision, dental problems, drowsiness, slurred speech, rashes, abnormalities in the blood and confusion. It is very difficult to get through life when you are challenged with these side effects. Sometimes they emerge immediately and sometimes the medication builds up in your body over time and you start to experience them sporadically. Either way, you aren't becoming healthier by taking the medication; you are simply accepting life with a different affliction.

In addition to improving your own health, coming off medication and relying on your own body's ability to heal itself will help the nation as a whole lower medical costs. The President of the United States, President Obama, has proposed a very complicated medical plan that will extend medical coverage to all Americans. This is great for the economy of the pharmaceutical companies and some medical professionals, but for the general public, it encourages a reliance on Western medicine and drugs. Pharmaceutical drugs do not promote healing as much as we give them credit for. They do reduce some symptoms and can aid in fighting off diseases, but the overall side effects of prescription medication often do more damage than good. Eliminating your dependence on these drugs for your own health and encouraging other people to eliminate their dependence will help to lower the insurance costs. I find it very sad when I read about my friend who has been told that she will be on a cancer medication for the rest of her life. The chemotherapy doesn't make her feel good, and leaves her drained. Her productivity is reduced, thanks to this drug. She is relying on the drug for her health and not enhancing her body's ability to heal itself. Meanwhile, the insurance premiums have to go up because more people are being prescribed expensive therapies such as these. Epilepsy and seizures, like any chronic illness, are not cheap. Your out-of-pocket expense is not the only one that is impacted.

5 CREATING A PLAN TO TREAT SEIZURES NATURALLY

Taking medication is definitely something that requires careful consideration. However, in addition to medication, or in place of medication, we need to optimize our own health and do things that will improve our health naturally. This will help us live a better life and end the reliance and dependence on prescription medication. Keep in mind that you are creating a plan for optimal health, not simply to treat your seizures. You will want to dedicate a good chunk of time every single day to improving your health. If you currently take medication in the morning and the evening, start to think about your exercise program and do it as religiously as you would take your pills. The benefits of exercise are that they reduce your breathing for a few hours after exercise. Try to make time for exercise twice a day. Your breathing exercises should be done throughout the day, whenever you can squeeze them in.

Telling Your Doctor

When creating a plan that implements natural alternatives, there are a few things that you should know about. Most likely, your neurologist won't approve or will offer little support. My doctor laughed at me when I told him that I was going to an acupuncturist. He said it wouldn't do anything. He encouraged me to stay on my medication. In fact, you do need to be careful what you share with your neurologist. When I came off medication, my neurologist told me that he couldn't work with me unless I would take medication, and he referred me to someone else.

Most neurologists are going to act like my doctor did. Most of them will tell you not to come off medication. They trust the medication, but naturally, they aren't living with the side effects on a day-to-day basis. A doctor's education is in pharmaceutical drugs. They study the chemistry behind them. They read the published studies by the drug companies and they trust the medication. Doctors are biased toward medication. They are unlikely to create a health plan that includes natural alternatives. However, this doesn't mean that the natural remedies don't work or that you shouldn't try them. The good news is that you can implement the

strategies for prevention without permission from your
doctor because they are simple to use.

Trying Alternative Medical Practitioners

Before connecting the link between
hyperventilation and seizures, I tried everything under
the sun. I started by testing out natural prevention
strategies with acupuncture when I was in California. It
didn't prevent seizures, and I continued to take
medication while I was trying the acupuncture. I'm not
entirely sure how acupuncture works, but it is very
relaxing and can help your body heal. The two
acupuncturists that I saw warned that acupuncture
wouldn't eliminate seizures, but may help them improve.
When I was in California, I did have a seizure on a day
that I had acupuncture, so I'm not relying on
acupuncture for my seizure control.

I tried chiropractic, which is a wonderful alternative.
I think the main place where chiropractic falls short in
treating seizures is that it takes a long time and they
don't teach you normal breathing techniques.
Chiropractic can help you gain better posture, which is
essential for the diaphragmatic breathing that is
important in oxygenating the body. For someone who is
suffering from a kyphosis (abnormal upper body front-
to-back curve in the spine) like I did, it will take a while
before your posture gets better. Diaphragmatic

breathing and having a straight spine go hand in hand. Neglecting to teach the diaphragmatic breathing means that the old chest-breathing habit will eventually kick in and you will become susceptible to seizures once again. Diaphragmatic breathing prevents slouching though, so once you learn how to do it, your posture will naturally improve. Chiropractic care probably contributed to my improvement, but it certainly didn't stop the seizures.

Trying Diets and Supplements

As I was testing out acupuncture, I also read a book called, *The Coconut Oil Miracle*. I tried taking coconut oil after reading online testimonials and discovering what a miracle cure it can be. The coconut oil alone won't prevent seizures. For some people, it is their miracle cure, but it wasn't a cure for me. I like to think that it made me healthier. I certainly discovered that it was tasty and fun to cook with. When I was on the Modified Atkins Diet for Seizures, I was taking 6 tablespoons of it a day as recommended by a holistic physician. I had a seizure despite the Coconut Oil and the Modified Atkins Diet, so I concluded that the key to my seizure control wasn't in my diet.

Diets were another thing that I tried in my pursuit of optimal health. One day I read about a raw food diet. It sounded so amazing that I went 'raw' for a month. I did have a seizure that month, so I moved on to the Gut and Psychology Syndrome Diet, or GAPS. Natasha Campbell-McBride is a neurologist who treated her child

with autism through the use of nutrition. I was sold on
what she had to say. The connection that she made
between seizures and digestion made a lot of sense. I
still had seizures on the GAPS diet. I stayed on that for
eight months and had three seizures before deciding it
wasn't working for me. It was also Christmas time and I
was heavily inundated by carbohydrate temptations.
After months of being so strict and having a couple of
seizures regardless, I gave into the holiday temptations
and started having a few extra carbohydrates. Around
this time, I discovered the normalbreathing.com website
where they linked the cause of seizures to
hyperventilation with the research studies to prove it.

When I realized that hyperventilation was the main
cause of my seizures after reading Artour's website
normalbreathing.com, something clicked for me. He
was describing my seizure patterns. Most of them
occurred between the hours of 4am-7am. Sleep
deprivation was a common factor in many, but not all of
my seizures. He talked about how hyperventilation
contributes to seizure control. This actually made sense
to me. While I had been a swimmer in high school, I
had good seizure control. When my doctor felt like
"maybe we should see if she has outgrown the seizures",
I had gone back to college, stopped exercising and was
eating poorly in the dorms. It is no wonder when he
took me off medication at that time that the seizures
returned. I wasn't exercising and my breathing was not
normal. I was quickly put back on medication and they
determined that I didn't outgrow my seizures and I

would be on medication for life. Now, with the knowledge of hyperventilation causing seizures, I realize that I hadn't addressed the cause at all. I was probably deep breathing during sleep and I definitely was overeating in the cafeteria since I had gained the "freshman fifteen."

I had been content to stay on medication for many years. In fact, I think I would still be on it if I hadn't lost my hair to alopecia and desperately wanted to get it back. I strongly feel that it is partly due to the fact that I took a lot of medication, which made my body susceptible to the autoimmune disease, alopecia. I know my hair will come back once my health is in order. I'm already seeing a few hairs return. I tried a variety of things before I found the one that is working for me. Creating a prevention plan for seizures for myself involved a lot of trial and error and reading on the internet. I started finding other people who suffered from a similar type of epilepsy and what they found to be helpful.

I started implementing the recommended breathing techniques and my seizures diminished in length from 60 seconds to 15 seconds. This was a huge breakthrough for me. It was the difference between taking hours to recover and taking minutes to recover. As I continued to practice the BreathSlim breathing exercises and increase the amount of time between breaths, I realized that I was getting healthier. My seizures were spaced farther apart.

Addressing Hyperventilation in Your Life

Many people assume that they are breathing correctly. However, if you are having seizures, it is unlikely that you are breathing correctly. You have become accustomed to a certain level of health and a type of breathing that is less effective. That is the reason that you are susceptible to seizures. I assumed that since I was a swimmer, I was breathing correctly. When I started breathing slower using the Buteyko breathing exercises and the BreathSlim device, I noticed an increase in energy and overall well being.

Changing a few things in your lifestyle will greatly enhance your seizure control and help you to feel empowered. First and foremost, you will want to ensure that you never hyperventilate. You want to retrain your body to breathe slowly, and in doing so your brain will get the right amount of carbon dioxide and oxygen. Carbon dioxide is calming to the brain. It helps to neutralize seizures. Oxygen helps your brain function properly.

When an organ is deprived of oxygen, it can become cancerous, become dysfunctional and die. Seizures are an indication that your brain isn't getting the right amount of oxygen and carbon dioxide, and you have too many excess electrons in your body. Seizures let you know that your body isn't functioning correctly and you need to address the underlying conditions. For people who are overweight, an expanding midline lets them know that they need to start exercising and eating right.

41

For people with epilepsy, a seizure shouldn't be an indication that you need more medication. Your body has an amazing ability to heal itself. It is your indication that you need to increase your prevention efforts. More medication simply covers up the symptoms. It covers up the feedback that your body is giving you to change how you are living.

There are things that will trigger hyperventilation. One of them is being overheated. I had a few seizures right after I'd had a hot bath. I also had a tendency to experience an aura without a seizure following it after coming out of a hot shower. Heat is going to raise your body temperature, and that can trigger hyperventilation. Now, I know to take cold showers and slow down my breathing.

Change the conditions and you will change your seizure control. While it sounds simple, you actually need to start implementing the changes in your life; and that takes time and effort. Set a goal to make these daily changes for 100 days and then evaluate your seizure control. Expect to become seizure free in six months, not one or two. Please don't feel that just because you have been doing something for 30 days that you will be better. Your body takes time to heal and change. If it were an overnight process, then we wouldn't have so many neurologists and medications available. The fact of the matter is that many people don't want to take the necessary action to improve their health. We like instant results, and prescription drugs offer that; which is why we rely so heavily on them. The other thing is that we often miss doing something that is important and that is when we don't see the results that we want right away. The thing that most people are missing, in my personal opinion, is the correlation between breathing and health. It was two decades before I put two and two together with the EEG and hyperventilation. You can retrain your breathing and start to obtain an optimal health state. It takes effort, time and patience, but you will improve.

My goal in creating this book was to give people an understanding behind the idiopathic seizures and a method to reduce or eliminate them naturally. These simple lifestyle changes and prevention strategies will do just that for you. Be aware though, that until your breathing is in the normal range 24/7, you will still be at risk of having a seizure. Addressing hyperventilation should be your main focus before eliminating all other types of triggers because when you normalize your breathing, everything seems to improve. I first started noticing more energy and better thinking from the BreathSlim device. Be consistent and be patient. It may take as long as six months to get your breathing to a normal rate 24/7. You will also want to ensure that you are breathing through your nose and with your diaphragm.

Here is the routine that I currently implement in order to prevent seizures:

1. BreathSlim breathing device -1 hour per day
2. 45 minutes physical activity in the morning
3. 45 minutes physical activity in the evening
4. Cold showers or alternating hot/cold showers
5. Eat dinner early
6. Avoid overeating
7. StressEraser Usage
8. Connecting to the Earth

The BreathSlim breath training device is the method that I implement to get my breathing to a normal rate. It is the fastest and easiest way to improve your breathing. I did not see any weight loss from the BreathSlim training device; I think the reason for this is that my body was fairly close to its ideal weight and I started eating my favorite holiday foods when I started using the device. Some people will experience weight loss with the BreathSlim device. For me personally, it is easier to have a gadget around to remind me to do the exercises, so I thought it was a worthwhile purchase.

Breath retraining can also be done through the Buteyko breathing exercises. These are ideal if you want to do something proactive during the day. There are a few exercises that you can do while you are walking across a parking lot or standing in line. The more you work on breathing correctly, the better your health will get. This will help you to prevent seizures. *Close Your Mouth: Buteyko Clinic Handbook for Perfect Health* by Patrick McKeown is the book that I purchased to learn the breathing exercises that can be done throughout the day.

Physical activity is important in getting your breathing to the proper rate and ensuring that you don't have future seizures. On his normalbreathing.com website, Artour recommends running. Running is great exercise. However, I feel like it may not be the ideal choice for someone with epilepsy to start with; I have had seizures while running. Your body does start to hyperventilate during exercise and if you don't have good breathing during the rest of the day, any extra hyperventilation can trigger a seizure. The reason you want to include physical activity is that after exercise, your body adjusts and it lowers your breathing rate for hours afterward. Exercise makes your body more efficient by oxygenating it. However, you need to get to a point where you can handle exercise. For the first few months, you may want to incorporate simple, moderate exercise with the Buteyko breathing exercises or the BreathSlim device and then increase what you are doing.

As I planned out my prevention strategy, it occurred to me that I needed to exercise twice a day. Initially, I started doing the breathing exercises in the morning to prevent seizures that could occur because I had hyperventilated at night. Remember, the most common times for seizures to happen are between 4am-7am. This is due to hyperventilating during sleep, poor sleeping conditions, disrupted sleep from snoring, and overeating late at night, thus reducing the oxygen content in your brain. When you wake up and immediately practice slowed breathing exercises, you regain the oxygen content that was lost and you retrain your body to breathe better.

Exercising in the evening helps to ensure that you'll have restful sleep at night. It helps to make certain that your rate of breathing is close to normal, and prevents mouth breathing at night. Mouth breathing will lower the amount of oxygen that you have in your body. At night, it is easy to end up mouth breathing without knowing it. If you have exercised prior to bedtime, it will help you to have correct breathing at night.

Recommended Exercises

The exercise that I recommend starting with is simple walking. Try to incorporate a mile or two of walking everyday at the beginning. Walking is something that almost everyone can do and you can increase the duration as your health improves.

Rebounding on a trampoline or balance ball is the next exercise that I recommend. Jumping up and down is fairly simple and you can easily get off the trampoline if you start to feel an aura. I have had seizures by the side of the road when I ran across a busy street to a bus stop, and another time when I was running for exercise before I had learned about the breathing techniques. You want to be in a safe place if you are exercising hard and that may not be running through your neighborhood. Once you increase your health and have a long stretch of seizure free days, you can consider running longer distances. I recommend building your confidence through moderate exercise that should be near a safe place in case you do have a seizure.

There are many additional health benefits that come from rebounding on a trampoline. Some people have actually cured their cancer from rebounding every single day. While epilepsy isn't cancer, this is evidence that rebounding provides strong overall health benefits to your body.

Rebounding on a trampoline is a very efficient exercise because it provides an increased gravitational load, which will strengthen the musculoskeletal systems. It protects the joints from chronic fatigue and the impact delivered when you exercise on hard surfaces. Rebounding increases muscle tone and improves the efficiency with which your body burns carbohydrates. Rebounding also lowers the pulse rate and blood pressure.

Rebounding on a mini trampoline aids the lymphatic circulation by stimulating the millions of one-way valves in the lymphatic system. Stimulating the lymphatic system helps to circulate the oxygen more to the tissues. Increasing the oxygen and carbon dioxide flow to your brain improves your chances of staying disease free and seizure free.

Rebounding increases your capacity for respiration. It tends to reduce the height to which the arterial pressures rise during exertion. Rebounding decreases the time which blood pressure remains abnormal after severe activity. It also assists in rehabilitation of a heart problem. Rebounding will increase the functional activity of red bone marrow in the production of red blood cells. Rebounding improves your resting metabolic rate so that more calories are burned for hours after you exercise. Jumping up and down on a trampoline aids the movement of fluid in your body, thus helping muscle performance and lightening the load that is required of the heart.

Rebounding will decrease the volume of blood that is pooling in the veins of the cardiovascular system, which will prevent chronic edema. Because rebounding on a trampoline improves circulation, it encourages collateral circulation (the formation of new branch blood vessels that distribute blood to the heart) by increasing the capillary count in the muscles and decreasing the distance between the capillaries and the target cells. By strengthening the heart, rebounding helps it to work more efficiently. Because each beat is more powerful, rebounding allows the resting heart to beat less often. Each heartbeat is more powerful and sends out a greater surge of blood around the body to nourish its 60 trillion cells.

Because rebounding is circulating more of the body's fluid, it promotes tissue repair. Rebounding for longer than twenty minutes at a moderate intensity increases the mitochondria count within the muscle cells. This is essential to increase endurance.

Acidity in the brain is something that we want to be

aware of and cautious about since it has been reported to be a seizure trigger. Rebounding adds to the alkaline reserve of the body. Rebounding also improves the coordination between the proprioceptors in the joints, the transmission of nerve impulses to and from the brain and the transmission of nerve impulses and responsiveness of the muscle fibers.

Rebounding enhances digestion and elimination processes. If you have a food trigger, it may be due to poor digestion. Improving your digestion may help you to decrease the number of food triggers that you experience. Due to the increase of oxygen that rebounding provides, this allows for peak cell function and better absorption of nutritious foods.

Almost every exercise will improve your sleep; and rebounding is no different. It allows for deeper and easier relaxation and sleep. This is extremely important to people with epilepsy, as poor sleep is a main cause of seizures. Remember that the majority of seizures occur between 4 am-7 am because of hyperventilation during sleep. Ensuring that you have a restful night's sleep should be a top priority if you are suffering from a seizure disorder.

It is reported that rebounding results in better mental performance and keener learning processes. This should be important to everyone, but especially someone who is affected by seizures. The seizure medication slows down your mental performance and that will be noticeable at work or in your lessons at school.

My favorite benefit of rebounding is that it tends to slow down atrophy in the aging process. Rebounding on a trampoline has been reported to actually reverse, prevent or diminish the hardening of arteries. By conquering this disease, you will keep your mind alert, skin smooth, skeleton flexible, libido intact, kidneys functioning, liver detoxifying, blood circulating, enzyme systems alive and hold your memory intact. It will give you a sense of control and an improved self-image. This is vital to your happiness and success in life.

Since breathing and seizures are interrelated, getting your breathing under control should be your highest priority. Breathing is controlled by changes in the volume of the chest cavity brought about mainly by the muscular movement of the diaphragm. Repeated rebounding exercises accomplish more muscle movements of the diaphragm with the consequent chest expansion. This results in an increased capacity for respiration.

Finally, as though those reasons to rebound aren't enough, it fights fatigue. Rebounding will tone the glandular system through the increase in oxygenation and the movement of fluids. This increases the output of the thyroid gland, the pituitary gland and the adrenals. All of these glands help to restore energy. Believe it or not, rebounding also supplies a reserve of bodily strength and physical efficiency. You will have more energy and be able to accomplish more. I've noticed that I am getting more done and need less sleep than I did in the past.

When I was diagnosed with a seizure disorder, the doctor had me checked to see if my thyroid was working properly because often people with juvenile myoclonic epilepsy have hypothyroidism. It wasn't producing enough thyroid hormones and I did test in the low range. While I have no idea if the low thyroid activity actually triggered the seizures I was having as a teenager, my doctor and parents seemed to feel that there was a correlation. I had no other hypothyroid symptoms besides testing in the low range. It is worth noting that often when one system isn't functioning well, others aren't either. Improving your health in one area is a catalyst to getting your whole body functioning better. (http://www.evolutionhealth.com/rebounder/rebounding-benefits.htm)

Eat dinner early

This is a lifestyle change that may or may not make a lot of sense to some people. When you eat, your body has to use up more oxygen to properly digest the food. If you eat and then go to sleep immediately afterwards, your food is being digested and using up excess oxygen, but your body also is in a horizontal position, which makes it impossible to ensure that you aren't hyperventilating while you sleep. Eating stresses your body and you don't want to be doing that while you are sleeping.

Eating early will ward off digestive problems. If

you are falling asleep just after dinner, you aren't giving your body the two hours that it needs to digest food. Neelanjan Singh, Nutritionist with Heinz Nutri Life Clinic explains that many of your digestive issues can be fixed by eating an early meal. *"It is important to have an early dinner because if you have a late dinner the body does not have time to digest it well,"* says Neelanjana. *"You are going to be in the prone position soon where you lie down flat on the bed. That way the digestive track is not working at its optimal level."* With your body in a vertical position, digestion is better. Waiting until you are not bloated with food will improve your sleep and that will improve your seizure control.

Eating an early dinner reduces the possibility of gastrointestinal problems, as well as acidity. It is important to be mindful of the acidity in your body because that can contribute to seizures. Seizures need an acidic environment in order to occur. It isn't that eating dinner early is going to suddenly make you seizure free, it is going to reduce the body conditions that are conducive to seizures.

Cold Showers

There are many health benefits to taking cold showers, but the main one that will benefit someone with epilepsy is that it will deepen breathing. This happens because your body is trying to combat the stress of the shock of the cold water and the vasoconstriction that is occurring. Your body feels an overall need to respire to keep itself warm. This will open up the lungs similar to the way that physical exercise does, and results in a higher average intake of oxygen. You will notice when you start to take cold showers that you don't feel as tired during the day and have more endurance during sports.

Your immune system will be strengthened when you implement cold showers into your daily routine. Researchers believe that the increased metabolic rate that takes place when the body tries to warm itself activates the immune system and releases white blood cells in response.

Taking cold showers will improve your blood circulation; alternating between hot and cold water while showering is an easy way to improve your blood circulation. As your body is exposed to cold water the arteries and veins constrict, or tighten. This vasoconstriction helps the blood to flow at a higher pressure because there is now less space for the blood to flow. This results in improved circulation. Your body has a natural tendency when exposed to cold to rapidly circulate blood to your vital organs to keep them warm. This increases the overall circulation. Having good circulation will ensure that oxygen is getting to your brain. Having the right amount of oxygen will help prevent seizures.

Your body's temperature will be lowered. Cold showers create a gentle form of stress that leads to thermogenesis, or your body's production of heat. This will activate the body's repair systems.

For those of you struggling with weight loss, you'll be happy to discover that a simple cold shower can increase your metabolism. Brown fat is heavily involved in burning energy. Being exposed to cold will naturally stimulate the production of brown fats. These are the cells that burn glucose to try to produce as much heat energy as possible. Having a higher amount of brown fat leads to more energy being burned per second and therefore, more weight lost. By increasing the brown fat, blood pressure and body temperature, chemical reactions in the body will happen faster than they would normally without regular cold showers. More weight loss will be seen and more growth and repair of muscles and tissues will be seen.

Increasing the cold exposure to our skin has a stimulating effect on the brain's "blue spot," the main source of noradrenaline for our bodies. This is the chemical that might be used to help alleviate depression. Cold showering fights depression.

Taking cold showers will help improve your lymphatic system. The lymphatic system is a system of tubing separate from our blood vessels. It is responsible for taking the waste away from our cells as well as helping to fight off the pathogens. The lymph carries away waste products and white blood cells handle the infection. The lymph relies on the contraction of muscles. When you take a cold shower, it causes whole-body contraction and this works excellently with the lymphatic system, squeezing the lymph up through the body. When the lymphatic system is not working properly, the lymph pools in far away places like the feet.

If you haven't been sold on the health benefits coming from cold showering yet, there are more. Cold showering keeps skin and hair healthy. Many people are aware that hot water can cause dry skin and hair. On the other hand, cold water can make your hair shinier and your skin look healthier. I can't attest to the shinier hair as I lost mine before I started my cold shower regimen, but my skin looks much healthier. I'm noticing the fine lines start to diminish. Cold water tightens cuticles and pores. This can prevent them from becoming clogged and diminishes the appearance of acne. Cold water also helps your body detoxify, which results in squeezing the toxins and waste products out of the skin. This detoxification can help the skin look younger. Cold water closes the cuticle, which makes the hair stronger and prevents dirt from easily accumulating on the scalp.

Cold showering can improve your energy levels. A cold shower will give you an invigorated feeling. It will help you feel energized and shake off the lethargy from the previous night's sleep. The reason for this is that the heart starts to pump faster and there is a rush of blood through the body. There are not a lot of studies to support this claim, but many people swear that cold showers are a stress reducer.

For most people, you won't want to switch to an ice cold shower immediately. There is a way to do it to make it much more enjoyable. I discovered that having a cold shower after working out was a very refreshing way to get clean. You can start lowering the temperature of your shower by using a contrast showering method. Spend some time in warm water and turn the water cold for thirty seconds at a time. Eventually, you will discover that you not only tolerate, but start to enjoy the cooler temperature.

Sources:

http://www.ncbi.nlm.nih.gov/pubmed/8925815

http://www.ncbi.nlm.nih.gov/pubmed/17993252

Essentials of Anatomy & Physiology, Elaine Marieb

Eliminate Stress

The physiological impact that stress has on the body causes you to start to hyperventilate. Therefore, stress becomes a seizure trigger. I never noticed a lot of stress in my life, but I did find a way to eliminate the stress. The StressEraser is a cool little tool that gives you a visual display of how your heart rate is doing and it tells you when to breathe. http://amzn.to/ZX6S2g. When you get three dots, you are breathing at a rate that is six breaths a minute. That is well within the normal breathing zone and a great target to shoot for. The stress eraser is a biofeedback tool that can help you slow down your breathing and reduce stress. Find some time throughout your day to pull out this little gadget and lower your breathing. I used it along with the BreathSlim device to see what kind of difference using the BreathSlim device made. What I noticed was that the waves were larger and it was easier for me to get to the three dots, or breathing six breaths per minute, faster and more consistently with the BreathSlim device.

During my most recent EEG, I used the BreathSlim device in combination with the StressEraser for about 3 hours while I watched television. It was a twenty-four hour EEG, so I was hooked up to electrodes and told to stay as still as possible. When I realized that was a requirement for the EEG, I regretted signing up for it, but the amazing thing that happened was that breathing slowly and getting into a meditative state kept my EEG normal. I also had more energy on less sleep. I think that night I slept four hours. Now, the recommended amount of time for sleep is eight hours a night, but I wonder if this number is arbitrary. I wonder if that is just for average people who really aren't very healthy. The Buteyko people seem to think that once you achieve optimal health, with slower breathing and the right amount of oxygen flowing through your veins, you have more energy naturally and sleep less. So far, this has been my experience. Not only do I have more energy, but I sleep less. I haven't figured out what to do at 3 in the morning, but I am awake and alert. Sometimes, I just lie in bed and daydream because it is hard to believe that I am up in the middle of the night.

All of the above is my personal plan for preventing seizures. It is important to keep in mind that my seizures were typically one minute tonic clonic seizures. I didn't have them daily, but was susceptible to them. When I did have one during the day, it was unlikely that I'd have another one that day.

Artour Rakhimov's website, http://www.normalbreathing.com/d-seizures-treatment.php, has several recommendations for the treatment of seizures. He states that in order to eliminate seizures, you must address the carbon dioxide deficiency, the oxygen deficiency and the free electrons in the brain.

According to Artour Rakhimov, "*In order to stop or treat approaching seizures (at the onset of first signs of seizures), the adults should apply either grounding of the human body (Earthing) or the Buteyko Emergency Procedure (or the Buteyko reduced breathing exercise) that increases brain CO2 and O2 levels and helps to prevent most seizures that take place during day-time.*"

"*In relation to clinical remission or cure of epilepsy, having more than 20 s CP 24/7 is the first step in the natural prevention and treatment of seizures and epilepsy using breathing retraining techniques. Achievement of normal breathing parameters (40 s CP) and CO2/O2 levels in the brain is the main goal of the treatment of seizures. My experience suggests that over 30 s for the morning CP is sufficient to prevent any seizures.*"

On his website, CP is short for control pause, or the amount of time that your body pauses between each breath. I've found it difficult to measure control pause (CP) as I can't always tell if my body is straining for oxygen or if I am holding my breath too much. For this reason, I determined that it would be simpler to use the BreathSlim device regularly and exercise to increase my control pause and improve my overall health.

Monitoring your progress with the Buteyko breathing exercises involves seeing how much oxygen content is in your blood. You can do this by counting how long between breaths; Artour calls this a 'control pause' or CP. He created a table to demonstrate where you are with your health in relationship to seizure control:

Body-oxygen level	Symptoms of chronic hyperventilation in those adults and children who are genetically predisposed to seizures
1-5 s CP	Life-threatening type seizures (including status epilepticus, complex partial seizures, absence seizures or Petit mal, tonic seizures, clonic seizures, myoclonic seizures, atonic seizures, and tonic-clonic seizures or Grand mal) can occur at any moment of time due to severe degree of overbreathing.
5-10 s CP	Simple partial seizures and complex partial seizures and

absence seizures; more severe types of seizure can be triggered by any slight provocation that further intensifies breathing and reduces body oxygenation and the CP down to about 5 s or less

11-20 s CP   Myoclonic seizures, atonic seizures, and simple partial seizures or focal seizures; a more severe type of a seizure can be triggered by strong enough stress or lifestyle factors that further intensify breathing so that the CP drops to around 5 s; if the existing light or focal seizure involves the nerve cells that control the respiratory muscles or the cells of the breathing center, the seizure will always progress to a more severe type; especially with the transition to mouth breathing and/or chest breathing.

20-30 s CP   Seizures become more rare and shorter in duration, but still can be provoked by strong factors such as abnormal blood glucose levels, emotional stress, and others

30-40 s CP   Seizures are virtually impossible

provided that the patient does
not reduce their CP below 30 s

Over 40 s CP   Seizures are impossible

When I try to measure my control pause, it doesn't
seem easy because I'm unsure of when to breathe next
and whether or not I'm holding my breath too long.
After a week of using the BreathSlim device, I found my
seizures related to the 20-30 CP range. They were
shorter in duration! It says that they can still be
provoked by strong factors such as abnormal blood
glucose levels, emotional stress and other causes. The
first seizure that I am referring to was actually after
Thanksgiving. There was probably a higher than normal
blood glucose level after eating a big Thanksgiving meal
and some emotional stress from visiting relatives. I also
had one the day after Christmas when my nephews
disrupted my sleep and I ate more than normal. The fact
that the seizures that I had after starting this program
were shorter confirms to me that something is working.
I'm still working my way up to a high over 40 second
control pause, but it does take time to retrain your
breathing. I finally feel like I'm doing something that is
working to improve my seizure control and overall
health.

It would be easy to quit the exercises and say this
didn't work because I had a couple seizures, but my
family did notice a considerable shortening in the length

of my seizures. This didn't happen for me when I was on the Modified Atkins Diet for Seizures. When I was on the Modified Atkins Diet and had the seizure at the middle school, a co-worker told me it lasted for about a minute, which was the average for me. Interestingly enough, she told me that when I was seizing, I stopped breathing. I read somewhere that not breathing is your body's way to regulate itself and get the right amount of gas exchange going in your lungs. Getting my seizure length down to fifteen seconds seems like a huge accomplishment; especially since my recovery time was reduced to five minutes as opposed to a whole day staying in bed to recover.

In order to address the free electrons in our bodies, Artour Rakhimov, author of the site NormalBreathing.com, recommends grounding, or Earthing. Earthing means 'connecting to the earth'. The Earth apparently gives off positive electrons and they help to counter too many negative electrons. This is an interesting concept, and I'm not sure how much validity to give it. I did purchase a book on Earthing and do connect to the earth with a pad on my bed during the night. It seems awfully difficult to prove to me. I was a special education physical science teacher for a while, and I understand the concept of negative electrons matching up with positive electrons when there are too many. People with epilepsy do have too many electrical discharges. That is apparent on an EEG. It seems difficult to prove that the Earth's charges are positive and mine are negative; and that simply walking barefoot on the grass will help eliminate them. Sometimes, simple solutions are the best, though. It isn't something that is harmful if you do it and it doesn't cost any money to try. In the book, *Earthing The Most Important Health Discovery Ever?*, Clinton Ober, Stephen T. Sinatra, MD and Martin Zucker further explain how eliminating the excess electrons from your body will help eliminate inflammation and disease. I'm actually not sure if there is a lot of seizure prevention coming from connecting to the earth overnight. However, if that is the key to my seizure-free lifestyle, I would hate to neglect mentioning it to you. There are many people who swear by Earthing.

6 CHALLENGES THAT COME WITH EPILEPSY AND SEIZURES

I conducted an informal online survey to discover the biggest challenge for people with seizures.
Sometimes it isn't the seizure itself. For most of my life, seizures weren't a problem. The medication side effects were impacting my day-to-day life more than the seizures were. Epilepsy impacts our lives in more ways than simply during the one minute we are convulsing or unconscious. They impact the way that people interact with us. Epilepsy impacts our independence, as driving privileges are dependent on whether or not the doctor feels like it is safe to recommend driving, and the state requires a period of seizure free time before allowing you to drive. If you are like me, your employment is impacted by the slowed cognitive function.
Discrimination does happen. I have experienced it in my employment.

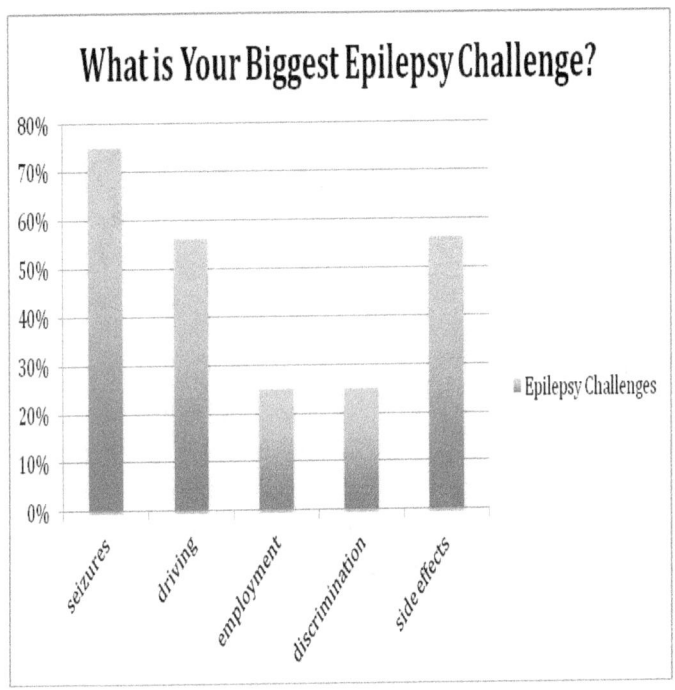

The medication side effects are daunting to overcome. For someone like me, I felt like I was resilient to the side effects. As a teenager, I was definitely in denial about being different. I felt "a little drowsy." Everyone else could tell that I functioned slower than the normal person. It wasn't until I was seeing double while I was driving that I realized there was a real problem with taking medication. It certainly kept me from having seizures, but I really don't think that driving while I was seeing double was a safe thing to do. However, when I initially started the car, I hadn't seen double in months. Logically, I should have been fine to drive.

The problem with being drowsy due to a medication is that it slows down your processing speed. This really affected my employment. I would think that I had understood everything that I was told to do, but in reality I was missing information. I was missing some directions. Multi-tasking was a huge struggle for me. I didn't realize that it was, because I just thought I was keeping up with the pace of everyone else. That was not the case at all. I was fired from my first job out of college at the Committee on Ways and Means after six weeks. They actually told me I wasn't doing a good job after four weeks and I tried to step things up, but I really didn't know what they were talking about; I felt I was doing everything they told me to do.

There are so many different side effects that a medication can produce that you may not realize that your medication is the cause unless it is one of the main ones and the doctor points it out to you. This is particularly true for people who are taking a newer medication. When I started having double vision from Lamictal, it hadn't been reported enough for a warning to be on the label that double vision was a side effect. The first thing that I did was go to my optometrist to get my eyes checked. I figured I needed new glasses anyway, and had no idea what was happening. It was a couple of years before the double vision reemerged and I knew could correlate the double vision with the anticonvulsants.

Seizures create a fear in people. The wonderful thing that I discovered as I started a business and started to get proactive about treating epilepsy is that action cures fear. When you start taking action in order to prevent the seizures, it helps eliminate fear. You begin to trust yourself; and that is really empowering.

There is an isolation that surrounds epilepsy. Most of your friends don't have to deal with epilepsy. The doctor can't refer you to other people who have it that are your age because of HIPAA laws, although if he is good he may refer you to a support group. I went to one of those as a teenager, but didn't feel like I could relate to the other people in the group. My seizures weren't so debilitating that I stayed home all day. I wasn't having a hundred a day, I was having them when I forgot to take my medication, so at the time I couldn't relate to the people in the group and didn't find it helpful at all. In fact, I found it kind of depressing because most of the people in the group just complained about their seizures and weren't looking for ways to improve their lives.

While I was writing this book, I discovered that connecting with other people who face epilepsy is a great way to give some validity towards your feelings and experiences with the disease. I found that this can be very therapeutic as I started connecting with people online who were sharing their experiences with epilepsy.

It was wonderful to see that I wasn't the only one who felt dependent because of my medication, and struggled with employment and discrimination. I also realized that some of the things that I struggled with were common to people who lived with this condition. It wasn't that I was absent-minded or lazy. The medication was slowing down my functioning.

The Epilepsy Blogger, Mandy Krzywonski, is great for encouraging conversations and discussing the impacts that seizures have on your life. She chose the epilepsy surgery and has a very positive outlook on her life. The following is an example of the type of discussions that occur online. It is wonderful to connect with other people who experience the same feelings and emotions that you feel. On this particular day, EpilepsyBlogger asked, "What is the biggest challenge that you face with epilepsy?" As you can see from this thread, many people with epilepsy face unique challenges that go beyond simply taking medication.

> Hope Elizabeth Welker - For me, it was always medication effects. I could never find one that gave me sufficient control without leaving me stoned and stupid.

> **Sheila Lentz** Sadie falls a lot when she is playing. She has seizures all day and when they happen a lot of times she looses her balance and falls. She has so many bumps and bruises and a few weeks ago, she was playing with her older sister and she had a seizure and fell face first on the side walk, scraped her little nose all up and bent her glasses

Lori Schneider My son Carter has,Lennox-
Gastaut Syndrome he seizures at least 100 times
or more a month; on his really bad days it has
been up to 100 a day ... this biggest problems he
faces is he cannot go to school and he cant read,
write or even count to 5, he will be 13 in
October, another problem is other children
where we live are cruel and wont play with
him... It is so bad that a 4-year-old on our street,
every time he sees Carter , says .. my mom said I
am not aloud to talk to you .... Oh my. This
breaks my heart ... p.s. I have been up all night;
Carter has had a grand mal seizure practically
every hour tonight ... sorry for ranting , but
thank u for letting me. Carter J. Ryon my son,
my hero xoxo

Stephen Piorkowski Mostly it's my
independence. I lost my right to drive. When I
lost my driving privileges I biked to work 40
miles every day. I feel sometimes as if I will be
punished every time a seizure occurs. Family
becomes traumatized and I feel that I hurt them.
I feel that I hurt them more than myself having
seizures. The people that love me watch me go
to extremes. I feel trapped and when I do I fight
to assert my independence.

Greg Collins Stephen Piorkowski, I agree

entirely!!!

Laurel Cook as a mom of 18 yr old son, be assured, no matter how much u think u hurt us we love u unconditionally and will do anything to help u!!!

Billy Ranney My independence, but that can be overcome! People lived 1000s of years without a car or other transportation. I feel a real anxiety in restaurants when I'm alone the noise really gets to me! I had epilepsy surgery 11 days ago so I'm really hoping that all changes.

Billy Ranney I also agree with Stephen Piorkowski I watch my wife and family go through hell every time I'm having a bad day or couple of days. They become care takers

Billy Ranney Our famous words as epileptics are "I'm fine"

Stephen Piorkowski F.I.N.E.(FEAR, INDEPENDENT, ANXIETY, EPILEPSY) sometimes I go through periods of Fear, I become more Isolated when I feel that I am dependant on people. I go to extremes to show that I'm INDEPENDENT, my ANXIETY of uncertainty causes stress and all of the above are the effects that EPILEPSY gives me.

Melinda Curle Stephen, I do the same thing! I hate feeling dependent.

Greg Collins in the process of proving my independence i have kept the ones i luv at a distance to protect them.

Billy Ranney Greg Collins I'm sorry that it has come to that for you! I hope one day you can open up to them and that they will understanding what you go through daily..

Jessica Keenan Smith Stephen Piorkowski I love the FINE acronym! I am working on another question for the Living Well With Epilepsy page more specific to stigma and I will work that in (if you don't mind me expanding on your idea!)

7 EPILEPSY AND EMPLOYMENT

Since one of the things that can trigger seizures is stress, you should carefully consider your employment status. For many people with epilepsy, it is a struggle to keep a job. For others, the stress of their job is contributing to their seizures. Transportation to your job can be a huge stress in your life regardless of whether you have driving privileges or not. When I would apply for jobs, I tried to make sure it was near public transit just in case I lost my license. This eliminated a lot of possible jobs in the suburbs without bus service. Another strategy that I used was that I would try to find a job and then try to move nearby so that I was living close to where I worked. What I didn't take into consideration was that I wouldn't be able to hold the job because my medication was slowing down my mental processing and I didn't realize that. It took me longer than the average person to process information. Often I would seem like an incompetent employee because I hadn't processed the third and fourth instruction that was given to me. I thought that I was working hard and was always confused by the comments that I was "lackadaisical" or "lazy." I certainly was trying my hardest to keep these jobs, but it was a struggle for me.

You may face discrimination on the job. I worked at a high school in Centreville, Virginia and one day I had a seizure there right before school started. I contacted the school to let them know that I was ok and I'd be in the next day. They actually told me that I couldn't come back without a doctor's note stating that I was fit to work. Well, that is fine and dandy if you can get in to see your neurologist quickly, but mine is so busy I usually have to wait a month to get an appointment. I was very disappointed and felt like this was an example of unknowing discrimination. I know that it is not county policy because as a substitute in another school, they were so nice to me and simply asked for an emergency contact in case it ever happened again. I haven't mentioned my seizure disorder to most of my employers because I felt like my seizure medications were working well enough and I shouldn't have a problem on the job. Notifying your employer can be tricky. It may be that they won't hire you because of the seizures and for some jobs involving heavy machinery that is understandable. However, I think that it is far more common that the side effects from the seizure medication impact your work performance and many people with epilepsy are let go because they are trying to get through the day drowsy or pushing through with double vision. I worked through a swimming shift with double vision once and it was awful; I was lucky and they needed swim instructors badly enough that they didn't fire me. I think that if I hadn't had such a great track record with the recreation center, they may have told me I was too much of a liability, but I had put in hundreds of hours without a complaint.

Getting a neuropsychological evaluation can help you immensely if you are struggling with employment. It can demonstrate to you where your weaknesses are and give you some ideas on what direction you should take with your career. I was shocked when I discovered that my processing speed was in the first percentile. I assumed that I was just like everyone else, but seizures and medication were slowing down my brain waves, as well as my cognition skills. I thought I could keep up with conversations and didn't realize that I was missing information when I spoke with people. While it made me feel better about losing the jobs, I still wished I had gotten a neuropsychological evaluation when I was first diagnosed. I had done one in my twenties, but felt like the examiner was rude, I was also in pain and uncomfortable, so I disregarded his findings. . It took losing a few more jobs to take note and really listen to the neuropsychologist.

I have taken it upon myself to start looking for ways to ensure that people with epilepsy can gain employment and can be successful. Eliminating the stigma behind seizures apparently takes a long time. There are employers who are not sympathetic to employees with seizures. Most of them don't understand that the seizure medication is causing delays in thought processes. I was fired from many of my jobs because I couldn't multitask very well. I didn't realize that they had asked me to do something and thought I was completing everything, but the reality was that I was missing some key tasks. The employers saw someone who was slower and didn't finish everything. As a teacher, I struggled because it required me to think about discipline and getting a message across. Either my discipline would fail or I wouldn't get the algebra content across. It was a rough two years that I spent as a teacher. Neither of them was successful because my discipline was lacking. Discipline requires a high degree of multi-tasking and thinking quickly on your feet. I was thinking slower and could really only focus on one thing at a time while I was on medication.

One job where I had lots of success was teaching swimming. For someone with seizures this is a pretty dangerous job. I didn't experience any discrimination at the recreation center because I had built up a reputation as a great volunteer and then a fantastic instructor. It was about eight years before epilepsy had an impact on that fun, part-time job. One day when I had just finished teaching, I started to see double. I went into the guard's office and sat down. My head was spinning, but I had experienced this before and told everyone that I would be fine in a little while. I was experiencing a bout of vertigo and double vision. It had happened before at home. I could see the fear on my co-workers faces and they later told me that my eyes were shaky. Luckily, all my students had gone home for the day. My employer was kind enough to allow me to wait out the scary side effects before driving home. I feel that because I had built up my reputation, there were no consequences to my employment. I was able to continue teaching swimming the next week. Unfortunately, that isn't the case for everyone. Often if employers think that they will have to make huge accommodations for someone with a disability, they will chose a different candidate.

It took me years to embrace the idea of entrepreneurship. I knew that a home-based business would eliminate the need for transportation and that would eradicate one of my major stresses in life – getting around after a seizure. However, for someone with epilepsy, self-employment is complicated by the pre-existing health condition clause. Obtaining health insurance without a major company is extremely expensive, and in some cases unobtainable. Purchasing medication and paying for ambulance rides that you don't need is difficult without insurance, so there was always the insurance factor hanging over my head when I was selecting employment. As long as you are drug dependent and having seizures, getting health insurance is going to be a headache. Living without it seems risky.

After a decade of spotty employment, discrimination from employers, and a neuropsychological evaluation that pointed out a processing deficiency, I decided that it was time to check out what kind of help the government offered. Let's just say it isn't much. While you can easily get a Schedule A letter and start applying for government employment, they really don't try to hire people with disabilities as much as they claim. I spent a year applying for those "set aside" positions. The reality is that they end up filling them with anybody. I didn't even get interviews for those positions; and I applied to hundreds of them. Many of the positions, I was overqualified for, but I applied for them anyway because I desperately wanted to secure the health benefits that came from government work.

Since the government didn't really help with employment, I read through my neuropsychologist report and embraced the recommendation of medical billing and coding. Medical billing and coding can be done in a quiet room, at your own pace and it does not require complicated decision-making. I was encouraged to try this type of employment. The nice thing about medical billing is that it can be done at your own home during flexible hours. If you happen to have a seizure in the morning, you can sleep it off and complete the work later in the day from your own home. This seemed ideal to me. Not having to travel to work and worry about transportation was a great relief to someone whose driving privileges were on hold until the seizure free period was met.

I realize that not everyone with seizures is going to have an affinity for medical billing. Not everyone will have the money that I had to invest to start my medical billing business. While I was networking with someone from my Business Networking International group, he commented that after retiring he set up his AFLAC business for a $400 investment. Another BNI member set up her network marketing company for roughly $400 and is making a monthly residual income of $2,000. I realized that for someone with seizures, this is a small investment for a business that can help you financially whether you are simply interested in part time work, need a full time job, or want a safety net for those times when the economy is down and you are looking for work or unexpectedly get fired due to a seizure at work. I set up a website to get started with my experiment in network marketing to see if I could do it. I knew a few people who were extremely successful with network marketing and I started learning from them. I also discovered that I can generate leads online, which is such a valuable skill when your transportation gets eliminated due to seizures. You must put forth quite a bit of effort learning the skills required to succeed; and expect to work hard, but in the end it pays off. Unfortunately, it isn't going to generate a huge income immediately unless you already are a great salesperson and have a large network. If you are used to hourly wages, it is a tough transition, but one that can pay off immensely. In this book, I simply wanted to provide some solutions for people who are strapped for transportation and struggling with their employment.

8 EXPERIENCES WITH DRIVING

I was one of those people who were lucky enough to get their seizures under control in time to get my driving license at age 16. My medication was working and I thought life was great. I drove my brother to high school and drove myself to swim practice. Once I took the car and drove half-way around the beltway with a friend of mine because I was lost. I was an okay teenage driver. I didn't have any major collisions. I do remember putting the car in reverse in the Oakton High School parking lot and going up on the curb during Driver's Ed. It took me a while to get used to directions and spatial awareness, but I doubt that had anything to do with my epilepsy. I wouldn't have ever considered changing my epilepsy treatment because at the time I was able to drive and that meant freedom. In my mind, my driver's license was at risk if I changed what I was taking. I didn't know of any other way to prevent seizures other than medication.

As a teenager, I was a people pleaser. In some ways I had to be to obtain my driver's license. I had to do what the doctor told me to do and report to the DMV. But watching the doctor react to the news that I had a seizure was always devastating to me. I felt like I let down my family and friends. They would be so proud of me for not having a seizure that when I had one I felt like a failure; and I didn't know anything that would control the seizures other than medication. After the seizure, I would lose my license and become dependent on them for the next six months or more while I tried to regain seizure control, something that I really didn't have control over while I was trusting that medication would address the problem.

A medication change will ultimately put your license in jeopardy. I think had I stuck with the high doses of Tegretol and Depakote, I would have kept my license this entire time. I was very heavily medicated and had great seizure control. On the other hand, I probably would have been broke because the doctors wouldn't prescribe the generic drug for someone with seizures – and those medications were extremely expensive. I also had no idea how drowsy I really was until I came off the medication. After switching from Tegretol and Depakote to Lamictal, I spent two days absolutely wired and didn't sleep as my body adjusted. When I questioned my mother about the drowsiness after I switched medication she commented, "You would talk slower and walk slower. Everything you did was slower." I'm glad she kept that to herself for the eight years that I was on both medications. The combination of medications allowed me to drive, but switching put my driving privileges on hold.

I changed medication when I was 22 because the Depakote and Tegretol that I was on at the time wouldn't have allowed me to have children and I wanted that option. Mostly, I was enticed by the idea of taking one medication instead of two. My doctor also informed me of a new medication that didn't have side effects. One drug instead of two with fewer side effects was so exciting to me even if I didn't think I was experiencing side effects. So, I chose to switch medication.

Switching drugs is a time period when you absolutely should lose your license. I don't care if the doctor thinks it is a great idea to sign off on your driving privileges or not, in my opinion, during the change it is worth taking a break from driving. For some odd reason my doctor allowed me to drive for the few days following the week I spent in the hospital while they changed my medication to Lamictal. I didn't drive for long, though, as a week later I had my first seizure on Lamictal. They just increased the dose a few more times until I was at a high enough level to prevent seizures. I was 22 and felt like that was pretty normal. It didn't bother me too much and before long I had my driver's license back. In retrospect, I don't think my doctor should have allowed me to drive at all during the transition.

New medications mean different side effects and unreported side effects. While I hadn't anticipated that double vision would happen due to my new medication, it showed up unexpectedly a number of times. There were a handful of times that I would be driving and suddenly see double. Now I realize how dangerous this could have been had I not known the roads and been pretty close to home anyway. My doctor would always sign off on my driving privileges if I had been seizure free and was following the medication regimen that he prescribed. He didn't really seem to mind that I complained about the double vision. It seems to me that if you have to pass a vision test to drive, your doctor should make sure you aren't seeing two of everything before signing off on your driving privileges.

Taking a break from driving for six months after a seizure seems like a fine way to keep the roads safe, but people with seizures aren't necessarily safer. I don't think someone who is having seizures should be operating a vehicle and absolutely agree with the law. While keeping people with epilepsy off the roads keeps other people safe, it does not keep people with epilepsy safe. I lived in a cute little apartment in Pentagon City for a while. I decided to focus on personal training and while I was en route to a training session, I ran across a busy road to catch the bus. Once I arrived at the bus stop, I bent over to catch my breath and started to feel funny. The next thing that I knew, I was in the ambulance. I had a seizure by the side of a really busy road. I could have easily been killed if the seizure happened moments earlier while I was crossing the street.

Despite my seizure at the bus stop, the bus is probably the safest and least expensive mode of transportation for someone with seizures. It is important to know that people with epilepsy are entitled to reduced bus fare. During my twenties, my doctor would either sign off on my driving license privileges or he would sign off on a document that let the Metro area transit know that I had a seizure condition. The doctor drove me nuts because he would always put that my condition was temporary. This last time he marked that it was permanent, and now I have a five year Metrocard that says I am disabled and get reduced fares, which saves me from a trip downtown to renew the disability card. Usually I would prefer not to be labeled disabled, but when they restrict your driving privileges, I think it is fair to get reduced fares. If you do have a doctor signing off on the reduced fare form, make sure you ask him to mark that your seizures aren't temporary.

Getting around without a license is tough. Everyone that I know approaches it in different ways. I interacted with Stephen Piorkowitz on Facebook. He rides his bicycle 40 miles to and from work. That is amazing to me. Not all of us have the ability to do that. Some of us need to project a professional appearance at work – and riding a bicycle isn't conducive to that. Weather conditions make biking possible in warmer climates such as California; I rode my bicycle to a tutoring job that I had in California. One day, I fell off my bicycle and cut up my hand pretty badly just as I was arriving at work. The kids I tutored really didn't want to see a bloody hand while figuring out math problems. These are things to take into consideration when you are selecting a mode of transportation.

My best advice to anyone who struggles with seizure control is to embrace walking as a method of transportation. The health benefits that come from walking are abundant. It is a way to squeeze an extra bit of fitness in throughout the day and that will help you prevent seizures as long as you practice nasal, diaphragmatic breathing while you are walking.

Since driving isn't currently an option for me as my doctor refuses to sign off unless I'm taking medication, I am relying on the generosity of others, walking and taking the bus. Suburbs don't typically have public transit to every place that you want to go and don't always have sidewalks everywhere you want to go, either. It can get really frustrating when the location where you want to be doesn't have easy access. Tyson's Corner in Northern Virginia is a hotbed of social activity and business, but it is not walker friendly. It also doesn't have that much public transportation going to and from the location, either. Taking a cab is more convenient, but the cost of cab rides adds up quickly. I'm extremely grateful for everyone who has given me a ride and the public transit system that allows me to get places.

9 THE ELECTROENCEPHALOGRAM TEST (EEG)

Regardless of whether or not you are taking medication or treating your condition naturally, a doctor will always recommend an electroencephalogram. I want to share my experience with EEGs with everyone because they are something that my family and friends don't understand and haven't experienced.

An EEG will let you know how often your brain is firing off abnormal electrical discharges. Too many abnormal electrical discharges and you will experience a seizure. Electrodes are attached to your head with glue and a computer monitors the electrical activity in your brain. There are a few different types of EEGs that are performed. The two types that I have had are the 24 hour EEG and the sleep deprived morning EEG. The 24 hour EEG allows you to walk around wired up to a small device that records your brain waves. The sleep deprived EEG is an hour long and you are lying down the entire time hooked up to a computer.

Most of the EEGs that I have done were sleep-deprived hour long EEGs in the doctor's office. The hardest part of those EEGs for me was staying up until two in the morning. I was already really medicated and usually slept about nine hours a night. Watching television to stay awake in the evening didn't really work because I would always start to nod off. The worst thing about those EEGs was picking the dried glue out of my hair the next day. I swear that they used super glue because I would be pulling that stuff off my scalp and clumps of hair would come off as well. The glue has improved a little bit since 1989 when I had my first EEG, but it still smells toxic.

While I was chatting with the technician during my most recent EEG, I realized that the test isn't necessarily the great measure of your brain waves that I thought it was. The technician informed me that even people who don't have seizures sometimes have abnormal brain wave patterns. I suspect that this is because they have you hyperventilate at the beginning. They are trying to aggravate the seizure activity. It seems to me that with the intentional hyperventilation, there would be a lot of false positives with EEGs, but due to privacy laws, I can only speculate on that.

I have had about a dozen EEGs during my life and

often when the doctor reviewed them with me, he simply told me that they were normal. I was medicated and seizure free at the time, so I didn't question the results. Before getting another EEG, you should ask yourself, if someone with epilepsy can have a normal EEG and someone without epilepsy can demonstrate abnormal electrical activity, why am I getting this EEG done? For me, I chose to do it to find out if the natural prevention methods that I was doing were working. However, I'm hesitant to place any trust in the results knowing that the hyperventilation that they had me do just triggered the abnormal brain waves that I had worked so hard to eliminate. Also, knowing that people without seizures can exhibit abnormal brain wave patterns under those conditions makes me a little cautious of relying too heavily on the test.

An EEG is not cheap, either. My latest test came in at $1,033.55. Probably the worst and best part was that I hadn't met my $2,000 yearly deductible yet, so I received no help from the insurance company. This is a great accomplishment for me. I usually met that deductible within the first two or three months of the year just by purchasing medications to control epilepsy. This year, I didn't purchase any medications and only went to the doctor once before the EEG; and that was to schedule it out of curiosity. This test is not something that I ever plan on doing again and it was simply for my peace of mind this time around.

When I scheduled my EEG, my doctor wanted to do a 24-hour EEG to get a better picture of what was going on in my brain. He was aware that I had stopped taking my medication and was not experiencing seizures. When I questioned him as to what would happen if the EEG came out normal, he told me that he would recommend scheduling a weeklong EEG in the hospital. So basically, if my brain were functioning well, he would hospitalize me and search for some seizure activity. At some point, you have to realize that more testing isn't going to solve problems. I was at odds with my doctor on this one, but agreed to the 24 hour EEG for my own curiosity.

The day of my EEG, my technician explained to me all her decades of experience. She also gave me that tidbit that normal people can have abnormal electrical discharges during an EEG. This lessened my trust in the EEG, but I was already there. She started measuring my head in order to glue to electrodes to my scalp. The measuring part doesn't bother me, but marking my scalp has always hurt. They press down with something that feels like a crayon and make a mark to know where to place the electrodes. After that, they need to make your scalp a little abrasive. They rub some gritty stuff on your scalp. It feels like sand is being ground down into your head. Once your scalp has been prepared, the electrodes are glued on with toxic-smelling glue. This is the worst part of an EEG.

I was severely disappointed to learn from the technician that they wanted me sitting around all day. This would not be an accurate reflection of what I do during the day. I was disappointed that the EEG would

begin by erasing all my hard work to avoid
hyperventilation by starting me out hyperventilating and
then I was suppose to sit around so that they could read
my brain waves better. My whole seizure-prevention
strategy revolves around being active, getting your blood
flowing and getting more oxygen in the blood going to
your brain.

During my test, I played with my brand new
StressEraser and BreathSlim devices while I watched
television. I was supposed to keep very still. I decided
that I would watch how the BreathSlim device changed
the biofeedback from the StressEraser. I was pleasantly
surprised to see that the breathing was at an optimal rate
when I used the BreathSlim device. After a few hours of
sitting around recording my brain waves, I realized I had
a lot of energy.   That night, I slept really well, but
didn't need as much sleep to feel refreshed. I couldn't
wait for 2 pm the next day when my electrodes would
come off. I was tired of sitting around. My head had
been wrapped in an ACE bandage that was so tight it
was giving me a headache. Television wasn't cutting it
for me. I had seen more than enough episodes of Guy
Fieri's Diners, Drive-Ins and Dives and I was bored out
of my mind trying to sit still without moving. Usually
when I watch television, I try to squeeze in some
exercise but the directions were to not move unless I had
to during the EEG. I just wanted to take a shower and
get the glue off my head. The electrodes were attached
to cords that wrapped together and attached to a
computer monitor around my hip. They weighed my

head down like a ponytail that I had grown out to my feet. It also freaked me out a bit because the heavy pull on my neck reminded me of the first time I had a seizure and my neck was cocked in a funny position, so I was a little paranoid that I would end up breaking my seizure free streak doing the EEG.

Some doctors don't schedule that many EEGs. Some feel you should have one every couple years. I've seen both types of neurologists. Understand that the test does have its limitations. It can let you know how much electrical activity you have on average in your brain today. That doesn't mean that when circumstances change tomorrow you won't have a seizure. It may help a doctor identify where the majority of the excess electrical activity is located in the brain and let you know if you are a candidate for surgery.

10 MY EPILEPSY JOURNEY

I grew up in a Washington, D.C. suburb in Northern Virginia. Life was great. As a kid, I enjoyed watching television, swimming, and playing with the neighborhood kids. When I was in grade school, it seemed difficult for me to run. I knew a friend who had an inhaler and got out of gym occasionally because she had asthma. When I was in second grade, I was lagging behind the other kids on the track. I wheezed a lot and started experiencing allergies. In retrospect, from my knowledge of breathing and seizures, this was the start of my epilepsy developing. This was an indication that I was unhealthy as a child. It was another six years before I had my first seizure, but when I think about it, other things in my lifestyle were inhibiting optimal health. In fifth grade, they detected scoliosis. I was also much taller than my friends and had a habit of slouching to be able to hear conversations with them better. Slouching decreases your oxygen levels and prevents diaphragmatic breathing. Most people with epilepsy are chest breathers and thus not getting the proper amount of carbon dioxide and oxygen in the brain that they need. Long before my first seizure at age 13, I was lowering my body oxygen levels on an almost consistent basis.

My first seizure was a terrifying experience that I will never forget. I remember being outside playing with my neighbor and my brother. As I cocked my head up to look at something in the sky, I experienced a funny twitching in my neck that I couldn't control. I was actually aware of the twitching and the fact that I couldn't control it. I also experienced a surreal feeling like my head was light. (I've never taken drugs to get high, but one of my friends who has epilepsy described his aura as feeling 'high'.) That is really all that I can describe because after that point I was unconscious. I did walk back to the house, but my mind didn't record that. There is period after seizures where you are semi-alert. You are able to do things, but you don't have any recollection of them. After my first seizure, I remember waking up on the couch in our basement and my mother informing me that I had had a seizure. I was shocked. Later my younger brother told me that I landed in dog poop and got that in my hair. My mother tried to hide that fact from me, but my younger brother wasn't worried about sparing my feelings.

As I lay on the couch after hearing the news that I had a seizure, I remembered watching an episode of Different Strokes where they made fun of someone who

had seizures, but in the end they befriended him. I
assumed that no one really was that mean to someone
just because they had seizures. I never expected the
feelings and emotions that have come from having
epilepsy. I assumed that it wouldn't change my life that
much; I would just have to take medication. What I
didn't count on were the side effects, the discrimination
and the feelings of inadequacy that come when you don't
have control over your life for a few seconds.

My seizures started when I was in middle school.
They had a negative impact on my social life there.
When I was in middle school, trying to fit in with
everyone, I had a seizure in study hall. They called the
ambulance and I got a ride to the emergency room for
the non-emergency seizure. It was pretty cool to see the
inside of an ambulance the first time. When regained
consciousness, I had a nice chat with the EMT. The next
day, I went back to school and one of my best friends
came up to me and told me, "Did you hear, someone had
a seizure at school yesterday?" I was so devastated to
hear gossip about me going around. It wasn't like I
meant to have the seizure. When I went into the study
hall the following day, my teacher felt that it was
appropriate to have the class discuss the seizure with me.
They all told me that they were scared and worried. A
thirteen year old does not want to be the center of
attention for something that she can't control. I really
had no idea what happened. I was unconscious during
the grand mal seizure. Instead of making me feel good
that the other students cared, I felt responsible for

scaring them. They kept telling me how scary it was to watch. It would have been nice if the teacher asked me first if we could discuss the seizure. Keep in mind that I had no real recollection of what happened. I was unconscious. When I actually regained my awareness, I was out of the room headed to the hospital in an ambulance. The seizure erases your memories just before and after the event. Most of the seizures that I've had I don't remember.

The first two years that I had seizures were probably the worst. It was a guessing game with how much medication to give me. I started out with Depakote, but soon afterwards my doctors added Tegretol. With each seizure, the dosage was raised slightly until I was on 3000 mg of Depakote and 1500 mg of Tegretol. By age 15, everything seemed to settle down and the seizures were "under control." I was over-medicated, but I wasn't having seizures.

I continued as a competitive swimmer on the summer league and a winter swim team. My mother probably was really supportive and didn't ever let me know that she was required to watch the practices just in case I had a seizure. I didn't think much about her being up in the bleachers because a few other moms were there as well. In fact, I didn't think about my seizure disorder when I was swimming. I assumed that I would be fine. There was one time that I did have a seizure during practice. My mother noticed that I started swimming in circles in the middle of the lane. She got my coach's attention and they pulled me out of the water. My coach was so funny after that. He would constantly brag about saving my life.

When I started dating, I made the ultimate mistake of trying to size up the men and determine if they could handle the news that I had seizures. I also would try to figure out if they could financially afford someone with seizures. Seizures were draining me financially and I assumed that guys without jobs wouldn't be a good fit if something ever happened to me. If men weren't working for a big company with a sizable health insurance plan, I thought it probably wouldn't work out and didn't even give them a chance. This is a huge mistake because people shouldn't be viewed based on their jobs. Limiting my options made logical sense to me, but I probably missed out on a lot of opportunities. In the back of my mind, I worried too much about my health condition and less on connecting with men. I felt incredibly guilty that I was dependent on my folks for health insurance support when I lost jobs and I didn't want to transfer that burden over to someone who it would impose too much on. Now, I look back on it and realize how ridiculous and detrimental that approach was on my dating life. I hate to admit my mistakes, but most likely, someone else is doing the same thing and can learn from my mistakes.

I had some seizures at social activities and was embarrassed by them. Sometimes people would be thoughtful and come to talk to me afterwards, but sometimes it seemed that they would avoid me because they didn't know what to say. The older I got, the better it seemed people reacted to the seizures. I don't remember the circumstances surrounding seizures, so occasionally I will scare someone and they need to talk to me about it because they are so shaken up.

I also became very complacent when I didn't have a drivers license. This is unfortunate. I missed out on a lot of activities because I was too proud to ask people for rides. It was difficult for me because there were times when people tell me they were willing to give me rides and then when I asked for them, they told me that they couldn't. I took that rejection a little too personally. I also didn't want to burden other people with picking me up for activities, especially if they were in the city. I knew that it would take them a while to come out to the suburbs to get me. Ultimately, you have to decide to stop doing that. You have to break through embarrassment and accept that not driving is part of life and you may have to ask for rides and occasionally face rejection. Asking people for rides is still difficult for me and I prefer to assert my independence and walk or take the bus.

I read a lot of self-help books. I don't know why I like personal development so much, but I do. For Christmas in 2007, I got Kevin Trudeau's book, *Natural Cures They Don't Want You To Know About*. That was the book that really sparked an interest in natural healing. That was the book that ignited my belief that I could overcome epilepsy. The problem with his book is that he recommends too many things and many of them are expensive. I started trying a bunch of things Kevin

Trudeau recommended that didn't have the impact that I
wanted on my seizure control. I tried cod liver oil,
supplements, detox baths, magnetic mattress pads and
saunas as a way to reduce the seizures and kick the
prescription drug habit. Eventually, I set his
recommendations aside and searched the Internet for
more ideas on how to come off anticonvulsants.

In August 2012, I discovered a holistic medical
doctor who would work with me to help me off my
medication. Although he wasn't a neurologist, he was a
physician who had helped children that had seizures
come off medication. He recommended the Modified
Atkins Diet for Seizures. I did have some seizures
following his protocol. The thing that I learned from
doing that was that my seizures weren't tied to my diet.
I followed the Modified Atkins for Seizures pretty
strictly. For me, diet was not going to have the impact
that I needed on my seizure control.

Now I embrace the notion that your body can heal
itself. I strongly believe that your body wants to heal
and it has an amazing ability to do so. This belief had to
form in me after many years of being told that I would
be on anticonvulsants for the rest of my life. I listened
intently to what the doctors told me and believed them.
However, they aren't the ones suffering from seizures.
They know about drug cocktails and what will stop a
seizure, but they really don't realize how their comments
and their reactions impact people with seizures on an
emotional level. Medication apparently can stop working
for you, or your body adjusts to it and you need more to

achieve the same results.

After I gave up the Modified Atkins Diet for Seizures, I turned to the Internet and found the normalbreathing.com site. The explanation of the cause of seizures fit my life. I was having them mainly between 4am -7am. I started changing my breathing using the BreathSlim device and my seizure durations started decreasing from an average of 60 seconds to an average of 15 seconds. They also became more spaced out. I now was empowered! I wasn't guessing about a supplement that might work, like the coconut oil or the herbal tea. I knew that there was a correlation between how I breath and my seizures. Even the doctors are aware of the correlation between breathing and seizures. I could recognize that if I wasn't going to have a regular sleep pattern such as when I was out late on a date or eating much later than normal, I would be more susceptible to having a seizure. Being able to identify triggers is a huge key to your success in controlling seizures naturally or with medication. I'm still working my control pause up so that I can obtain optimal health. Right now, I'm close to breaking the 30 second CP (control pause). Once I get up to 40 seconds, seizures should be impossible! Even if they aren't impossible, I feel much healthier with my new exercise routine, my diaphragmatic breathing and healthy eating. Now I know I'm doing things that prevent seizures. Now I feel empowered.

I'm working on empowering other people with epilepsy. I created a website to help other people with epilepsy learn how to prevent seizures through natural methods and actually support themselves with network marketing because it is something that can be done from home and requires no transportation. Discrimination is low with network marketing companies and there are lots of companies to choose from. The business model is a little different, but you can be very successful with it. You can visit my website at melindacurle.com and learn more business tips to empower people with epilepsy.

I have started sharing my experiences with people through radio interviews to help not only raise epilepsy awareness, but also to inspire other people with epilepsy. For years, I assumed that epilepsy was something that simply couldn't be overcome, but cultivating that belief doesn't allow one to overcome it. I discovered that you must find the determination in yourself and believe that your body will heal before you will be able to heal.

This year was the year that I became much more determined. I determined that I would not rely on someone else for employment. I started Precision Revenue Services, a medical billing company as a way to earn money without worrying about whether or not I had transportation to get to work. Eliminating the medication lifted my spirits quite a lot. I started to think bigger and find solutions to problems. Previously, I could see a lot of road blocks and found it difficult to make plans. I still struggle with planning, but I'm finding that it actually is possible and I'm getting better at it everyday.

Eliminating medication from my daily life was an exercise in stepping outside my comfort zone. I was leaving the known path of taking medication for seizure control and exploring the unknown.

REFERENCES

http://www.ncbi.nlm.nih.gov/pubmed/8925815

http://www.ncbi.nlm.nih.gov/pubmed/17993252

Essentials of Anatomy & Physiology, Elaine Marieb

http://epilepsy.com/epilepsy/seizure_triggers

http://www.normalbreathing.com/d-seizure-threshold.php

Campbell-McBride, Natasha. Gut and Psychology
    Syndrome Natural Treatment for Dyspraxia,
    Autism, A.D.D., Dyslexia, A.D.H.D., Depression,
    Schizophrenia. Amersham, Buckinghamshire. 2010.
    Print.

Bonus

I really wanted to make it to the Amazon best seller list. As part of my book launch, I created some bonus material that you can find on http://melindacurle.com/bonus. There is a wonderful Facebook marketing course, a fun lead generation webinar and I'm providing a link to my Fitting Fitness In webinar that I'm having exclusively for people who purchased my book on the launch day. I will be sharing my tips and tricks for getting workouts in on the go and will share some of the recipes that I use on a daily basis.

www.ingramcontent.com/pod-product-compliance
Lightning Source LLC
Chambersburg PA
CBHW070540290526
45790CB00002B/572